PREDIABETES
A FUNDAMENTAL TEXT

Pathophysiology
Complications
Management
Reversal

Sam Dagogo-Jack, MD, DSc

American Diabetes Association®

Director, Book Operations, Victor Van Beuren; *Managing Editor, Books,* John Clark; *Associate Director, Book Marketing,* Annette Reape; *Acquisitions Editor,* Jaclyn Konich; *Design,* Jeska Horgan-Kobelski; *Production Services,* KnowledgeWorks Global, Ltd., *Printer,* Lightning Source.

Printed in the United States of America
1 3 5 7 9 10 8 6 4 2

The suggestions and information contained in this publication are generally consistent with the Standards of Medical Care in Diabetes and other policies of the American Diabetes Association, but they do not represent the policy or position of the Association or any of its boards or committees. Reasonable steps have been taken to ensure the accuracy of the information presented. However, the American Diabetes Association cannot ensure the safety or efficacy of any product or service described in this publication. Individuals are advised to consult a physician or other appropriate health care professional before undertaking any diet or exercise program or taking any medication referred to in this publication. Professionals must use and apply their own professional judgment, experience, and training and should not rely solely on the information contained in this publication before prescribing any diet, exercise, or medication. The American Diabetes Association—its officers, directors, employees, volunteers, and members—assumes no responsibility or liability for personal or other injury, loss, or damage that may result from the suggestions or information in this publication.

♾ The paper in this publication meets the requirements of the ANSI Standard Z39.48-1992 (permanence of paper).

American Diabetes Association titles may be purchased for business or promotional use or for special sales. To purchase more than 50 copies of this book at a discount, or for custom editions of this book with your logo, contact the American Diabetes Association at the address below or at booksales@diabetes.org.

American Diabetes Association
2451 Crystal Drive, Suite 900
Arlington, VA 22202

DOI: 10.2337/9781580407625

Library of Congress Control Number: 2021941961

Dedication

This book is dedicated to the physicians, scientists, nurses, dietitians, pharmacists, exercise physiologists, psychologists, lifestyle coaches, and all professional individuals and laypersons engaged in the research, discovery, dissemination, translation, application, and execution of the simple yet profound idea that modest lifestyle changes can help individuals at risk for type 2 diabetes avoid that diagnosis. Those individuals at high risk of type 2 diabetes have the condition known as prediabetes.

This book also is dedicated to the nearly 90 million people in the United States and 374 million worldwide who live with prediabetes, in the hopes that the information contained herein will provide them and their healthcare team the knowledge necessary for blocking the occurrence of diabetes, reversing prediabetes, and restoring normal glucose regulation.

Disclosures

Dr. Dagogo-Jack has served as a principal investigator or co-investigator for clinical trial contracts between the University of Tennessee and AstraZeneca, Novo Nordisk, and Boehringer-Ingelheim; has served as a consultant and advisory board member for AstraZeneca, Bayer, Boehringer-Ingelheim, Janssen Pharmaceuticals, Merck, Novo Nordisk, and Sanofi; and holds equity interests in Jana Care, Inc., and Aerami Therapeutics. He has also served as an expert for Sidley Austin, Adam and Reese, and Wheeler Trigg O'Donnell law firms on litigation related to diabetes and hormonal disorders.

Preface

Diabetes currently affects ~30 million adults in the United States and 463 million people worldwide. With the rare exception of neonatal diabetes, people with type 2 diabetes, which explains 90–95% of the diabetes burden, were born with normal glucose regulation and maintained that state for several years or decades before experiencing progressive deterioration in glucose regulation. The transition from normal glucose regulation to type 2 diabetes is punctuated by a variable interlude in an intermediate stage characterized by impaired fasting glucose and/or impaired glucose tolerance.

Prediabetes, the conventional term for the intermediate stage, is diagnosed by documenting impaired fasting glucose (fasting plasma glucose 100–125 mg/dL [5.5–6.9 mmol/L]) or impaired glucose tolerance (2-h postload plasma glucose 140–199 mg/dL [7.8–11.0 mmol/L] during oral glucose tolerance test) or an HbA_{1c} level of 5.7–6.4% (39–46 mmol/mol). Using those diagnostic criteria, nearly 90 million U.S. adults and more than 374 million people worldwide have prediabetes. Marked increases in the prevalence of diabetes and prediabetes over the next decade have been predicted. Diabetes exacts a huge economic and human toll as the leading cause of blindness, kidney disease, amputation, heart disease, and stroke.

Excellent glycemic control decreases the risks of diabetes complications; however, ~50% of people with diabetes worldwide achieve suboptimal glycemic control. Thus, along with improving glucose control in people with diabetes, the dominant strategy for stemming the epidemic is primary prevention. Based on the natural history of type 2 diabetes, intervention at the stage of prediabetes can interrupt development of full-blown disease. Therefore, focusing on prediabetes, is compelling. However, a deeper understanding of the pathobiology of prediabetes is critical to the discovery and delivery of programs for preventing diabetes. Numerous predictive risk factors have been identified for the initial escape from normal glucose regulation toward prediabetes and the subsequent transition to diabetes.

Focusing on prediabetes, this book first discusses the demographic, anthropometric, biobehavioral, and biochemical factors that drive the transition from normoglycemia to prediabetes. Emerging knowledge from genomics, transcriptomics, microRNAs, metabolomics, and microbiomics is incorporated into an expansive treatise on the pathobiology of prediabetes. People with persistent prediabetes are at increased risks for multiple vascular complications; the frequency of prediabetic microvascular and macrovascular complications and the mechanisms for their occurrence are discussed in detail.

Next, the focus shifts to evidence-based management of prediabetes and prevention of type 2 diabetes. Prediabetes either progresses to type 2 diabetes or remains persistent, seldom remitting spontaneously. Lifestyle modification and certain medications prevent progression from prediabetes to type 2 diabetes and may even induce remission of prediabetes in some people. Remission of prediabetes is desirable, because it is associated with long-term protection from future diabetes and its complications.

Finally, this book discusses how the strategies successfully used for diabetes prevention in landmark randomized, controlled clinical trials can be translated in communities around the world. Emphasis is given to practical adaptations that would enable the establishment of cost-effective community diabetes prevention initiatives.

The ideas discussed here are germane to developed and developing countries; low-, middle-, and high-income regions; and high- or low-literacy segments of the populace. Interventions using lifestyle modification are prioritized over medications, but novel approaches (including cyclical medication strategy, designer nutraceuticals, and metabolic surgery) are also discussed. Current lifestyle intervention protocols have been more effective at preventing progression from prediabetes to type 2 diabetes than they have been at restoring normal glucose regulation. This book makes the case that restoration of normal glucose regulation carries numerous benefits and should be the primary goal of intervention in people with prediabetes.

Contents

Chapter 1

Overview of the Epidemiology and Pathophysiology of Diabetes

Epidemiology of Diabetes

Diabetes describes a group of disorders of glucose metabolism characterized by hyperglycemia. Currently, diabetes is diagnosed if fasting plasma glucose is ≥7.0 mmol/L (126 mg/dL) or a 2-h plasma glucose is ≥11.1 mmol/L (200 mg/dL) during an oral glucose tolerance test. A hemoglobin A_{1c} (A1C) level of ≥6.5% can also be used to diagnose diabetes.[1] The U.S. Centers for Disease Control and Prevention (CDC) estimated that 34.2 million people of all ages in the United States (10.5%) had diabetes in 2018.[2] Of that number, 34.1 million were adults aged 18 years or older (13% of all U.S. adults). The prevalence of diabetes increased with age, with the highest burden seen in people aged 65 years or older, among whom 26.8% had diabetes.[2] The CDC also reported that 21.4% of adults with diabetes (7.3 million) were unaware of their diabetes status. Global estimates by the International Diabetes Federation in 2019 indicate that approximately 463 million adults currently have diabetes, and the number is projected to increase to 578 million adults by 2030 and 700 million by 2045.[3] Table 1.1 shows the list of the top 10 countries with the highest numbers of adults with diabetes in 2019 and projected data for 2045.

Diabetes is a global epidemic that now ranks among the leading noncommunicable public health challenges of the present era.[4,5] The number of people living with diabetes has increased by more than three-fold over the past 2 decades.[3–6] As the leading cause of blindness, amputation, and chronic kidney disease, and a major contributor to myocardial infarction, heart failure, stroke, and peripheral vascular disease, diabetes exerts a huge toll on quality of life and longevity.[7–10] Type 2 diabetes accounts for ~90–95% of the diabetes burden. Because of the largely asymptomatic nature of early type 2 diabetes, 21.4% of affected individuals in the United States are undiagnosed, and half of the 463 million people with diabetes worldwide are undiagnosed.[2,3] Such individuals with undiagnosed diabetes, nonetheless, remain at risk of developing diabetes complications. In many large studies, including the UK Prospective Diabetes Study, nearly one-quarter of people with newly diagnosed type 2 diabetes already have developed one or more complications.[11,12]

Table 1.1—Top 10 Countries With Current and Projected Number of Adults (20–79 Years of Age) With Diabetes

2019			2045		
Rank	**Country**	**Millions**	**Rank**	**Country**	**Millions**
1	China	116.4	1	China	147.2
2	India	77.0	2	India	134.2
3	United States	31.0	3	Pakistan	37.1
4	Pakistan	19.4	4	United States	36.0
5	Brazil	16.8	5	Brazil	26.0
6	Mexico	12.8	6	Mexico	22.3
7	Indonesia	10.7	7	Egypt	16.9
8	Germany	9.5	8	Indonesia	16.6
9	Egypt	8.9	9	Bangladesh	15.0
10	Bangladesh	8.4	10	Turkey	10.4

Adapted from the *IDF Diabetes Atlas.*[3]

Through its numerous complications and complexity of care, diabetes consumes an enormous proportion of the health care budget. Estimates by the American Diabetes Association show that the economic costs of diabetes in 2017 amounted to $327 billion (a 33% increase from the estimate of $245 billion in 2012).[13,14] The annual global direct costs of diabetes in 2019, as estimated by the International Diabetes Federation, amounted to $760 billion, and that amount is projected to increase to $825 billion by 2030 and to $845 billion by 2045.[3] Management of diabetes complications accounts for >50% of the huge costs. Indirect economic costs arising from disability, absenteeism, presentism, premature death, and other health-related negative impacts are estimated to add an additional 35% to the annual global direct health care expenditures associated with diabetes.[3] Most of the economic costs have been estimated using the adult population with diabetes. The increasing prevalence of diabetes (especially type 2 diabetes) among children and adolescents[15] and the additional costs over decades of life will undoubtedly further escalate the economic burden of diabetes in the future.

Pathophysiology of Diabetes

The two broad types of diabetes, type 1 diabetes and type 2 diabetes, have different underlying pathophysiological mechanisms. Type 1 diabetes accounts for 5–10% of the global diabetes burden, typically affects younger people, and is caused by absolute insulin deficiency. Autoimmune mechanisms directed at the pancreatic islet β-cells account for the loss of insulin secretion in almost all cases of type 1 diabetes. An interaction between inherited HLA haplotypes and putative environmental triggers initiates the autoimmune destruction of pancreatic islet β-cells that eventually leads to insulinopenia and development of hyperglycemia in individuals susceptible to type 1 diabetes. The interaction of genetic and environmental factors in the pathogenesis of type 1 diabetes has been studied in well-defined sets of monozygotic twins. The concordance rate of development of type 1 diabetes in an identical twin with an affected sibling is <50%.[16] As monozygotic or identical twins share 100% of their genes, the lack of 100% concordance in type 1 diabetes in the co-twin of a proband indicates that environmental factors (or posttranslational epigenetic factors) play a significant role in mediating susceptibility to type 1 diabetes. In support of the latter notion, the concordance rate of type 1 diabetes in monozygotic twins is higher if the twins are reared together than if reared apart. Furthermore, there is a time-dependent rapid decline in the rate of occurrence of type 1 diabetes in co-twins of affected twins in the years after diagnosis of the index twin, again consistent with an environmental mechanism.[16]

Type 2 diabetes usually affects older adults but is occurring with increasing frequency among children and adolescents. The strong genetic element in type 2 diabetes is indicated by a concordance rate of >90% in an identical twin of an affected sibling.[17,18] Insulin resistance (usually in association with obesity) and relative insulin deficiency are two key pathophysiological factors that lead to type 2 diabetes. Insulin resistance is necessary but not sufficient to induce type 2 diabetes, because the pancreatic β-cells are programmed to compensate by increasing insulin secretion to levels that can maintain normal blood glucose. Indeed, insulin secretion in amounts commensurate with insulin resistance (insulin demand) guarantees freedom from hyperglycemia. Therefore, it is the occurrence of combined insulin resistance and β-cell dysfunction (impaired insulin secretion) that permits type 2 diabetes to manifest.[19] Normally, the β-cells are programmed to expand in size and increase their insulin output to meet increased demands imposed by obesity or pregnancy[20]; however, such compensatory mechanisms are not evident in patients with diabetes.

Besides insulin resistance and β-cell dysfunction, current understanding recognizes multiple other pathophysiological defects in type 2 diabetes (Fig. 1.1). The list includes impaired postprandial glucagon suppression (α-cell dysfunction), increased lipolysis, exaggerated hepatic glucose production, incretin deficiency/resistance, maladaptive renal glucose reabsorption, and central nervous system defects (including impaired dopaminergic tone and dysregulation of appetite and satiety).[20,21] Insulin resistance can be inherited or acquired. Acquired forms of insulin resistance can be found in states of obesity, aging, physical inactivity, and consumption of high-fat, high-carbohydrate diets, among others.[22,23]

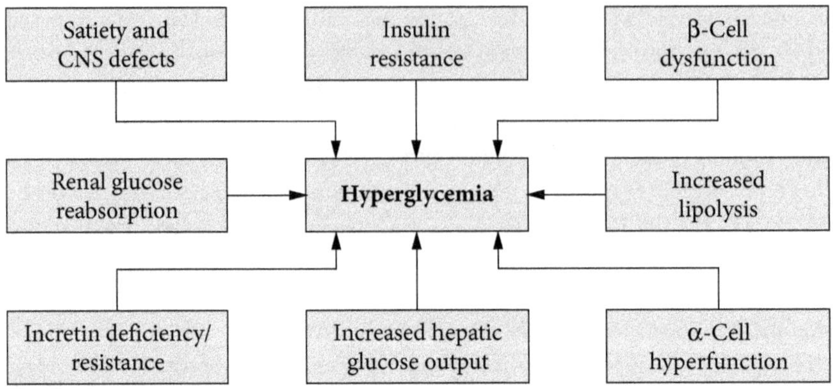

Figure 1.1—Pathophysiological defects in type 2 diabetes. CNS, central nervous system.

Dietary Fat and Carbohydrates

Diet-derived long-chain fatty acids are transported from the cytosol into mitochondria as long-chain fatty acids–coenzyme A (CoA) for β-oxidation. The outer and inner mitochondrial membrane shuttle enzymes, carnitine palmitoyl transferase (CPT)-1 and CPT-2, regulate the delivery of long-chain fatty acids into mitochondrial oxidation sites. Saturation or impairment of the shuttle process that leads to accumulation of long-chain fatty acids in the cytoplasm can result in lipotoxicity, cellular dysfunction, and cell death.[24] The intracellular accumulation of long-chain fatty acids along with diacylglycerol derived from intracellular glucose can activate certain isoforms of protein kinase C, leading to aberrant phosphorylation of the insulin receptor, impaired insulin signaling, and consequent insulin resistance.[25]

Acetyl-CoA, generated after glycolysis in the Krebs cycle, is converted to malonyl-CoA by the enzyme acetyl-CoA carboxylase. Malonyl-CoA is the activated two-carbon donor required for de novo lipogenesis. Malonyl-CoA also is an allosteric inhibitor of CPT-1, which blocks the transport and oxidation of fatty acids in mitochondria.[26,27] Glucose abundance also increases the formation of intracellular diacylglycerol. Thus, multiple metabolic pathways link intracellular glucose abundance (usually derived from carbohydrate consumption) to increased de novo lipogenesis, impaired fat oxidation, and accumulation of intracellular long-chain fatty acids, thereby increasing the risks of lipotoxicity and insulin resistance.[28,29] Remarkably, behavioral interventions such as calorie restriction (especially reduction of carbohydrate and fat intake), increased physical activity, and weight loss have a profound effect in ameliorating the insulin resistance induced by the aforementioned cellular and molecular mechanisms.[30–34]

Risk Factors for Diabetes

As for most chronic diseases, the development of diabetes involves genetic predisposition and environmental risk factors or triggers. In the case of type 1 diabetes, certain genes of the major histocompatibility complex have long been recognized as susceptibility factors.[1] Also, >60 variants across the human genome have been associated with increased risk of type 2 diabetes; however, the effect size of these individual gene variants is rather modest.[35–38] Aging and several other factors (including overweight/obesity, physical inactivity, history of gestational diabetes, hypertension, and dyslipidemia) have been associated with increased risk of type 2 diabetes.[1] These risk factors interact with genetic predisposition (indicated by a family history of diabetes and/or high-risk ethnic heritage) to induce glucose dysregulation and promote the development of diabetes. The interplay of genes and the environment was evident in the studies that showed a three-fold increase in the rate of type 2 diabetes in Japanese immigrants to the United States compared with native Japanese.[39]

The increasing rates of diabetes parallel those of overweight/obesity, which makes a prima facie case for weight gain as a leading culprit of the diabetes epidemic. However, type 2 diabetes is seen even among nonobese individuals, and a substantial proportion of overweight/obese people escape the diagnosis. These paradoxes indicate a current lack of complete understanding of the etiology of the modern diabetes pandemic. The recent dramatic increase in diabetes prevalence (more than three-fold in 20 years), which mirrors the trends in obesity rates, can hardly be explained by new genetic mutations and is more likely due to environmental factors. In a recent report from the Framingham Offspring Cohort,[40] participants who lived close to a major roadway (within 50 meters) had higher fasting plasma glucose levels than those who lived farther away (>400 meters). Among the same cohort, exposure to traffic-related air pollutants (fine particulate matter, black carbon, and nitrogen oxides) was associated with higher plasma glucose, independent of age or obesity status.[40] A direct association between exposure to fine particles and higher levels of glucose and insulin resistance has been shown in animal models.[41] Although the exact mechanisms linking proximity to major roadways to increased risk of dysglycemia in humans remain to be elucidated, exposure to fine particulate matter air pollutants is known to induce proinflammatory gene expression, altered chemokine profile, and systemic inflammation, manifested by elevated TNF-α and IL-6 levels in humans and animals.[41] Besides exposure to traffic-related gaseous pollutants, other conditions (including noise, sleep impairment, and psychological stress) associated with proximity to major highways could potentially affect glucose homeostasis. Some of the nontraditional or emerging risk factors believed to be contributing to the diabetes pandemic include the intrauterine environment, socioeconomic status, urbanization, the

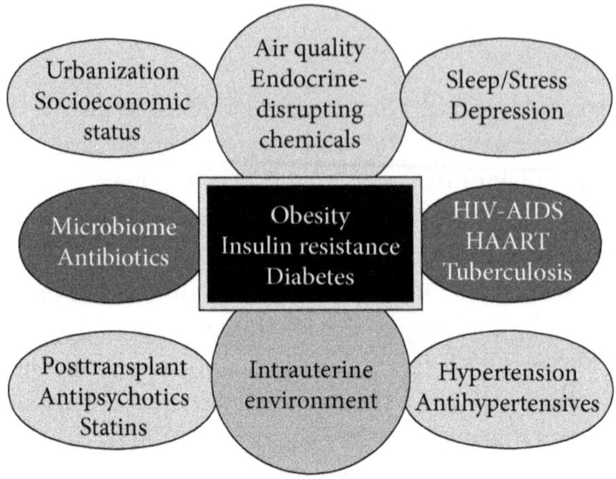

Figure 1.2—Nontraditional and emerging environmental risk factors for obesity and diabetes.

microbiome, endocrine-disrupting chemicals, air pollution, prescription and non-prescription medications, and sleep disorders (including sleep apnea, hyposomnia, and hypersomnia)[40–47] (Fig. 1.2).

References

1. American Diabetes Association. 2. Classification and diagnosis of diabetes: *Standards of Medical Care in Diabetes—2020. Diabetes Care* 2019; 43(Suppl. 1):S14–S31
2. Centers for Disease Control and Prevention. *National Diabetes Statistics Report, 2020. Estimates of Diabetes and Its Burden in the United States.* Atlanta, GA, Centers for Disease Control and Prevention, U.S. Department of Health and Human Services. Available from https://www.cdc.gov/diabetes/pdfs/data/statistics/national-diabetes-statistics-report.pdf. Accessed 28 October 2020
3. International Diabetes Federation. *IDF Diabetes Atlas*. 9th ed. Brussels, Belgium: International Diabetes Federation, 2019
4. World Health Organization. *Global Status Report on Noncommunicable Diseases 2016*. Geneva, World Health Org., 2016
5. Shaw JE, Sicree RA, Zimmet PZ. Global estimates of the prevalence of diabetes for 2010 and 2030. *Diabetes Res Clin Pract* 2010;87:4–14
6. Geiss LS, Wang J, Cheng YJ, et al. Prevalence and incidence trends for diagnosed diabetes among adults aged 20 to 79 years, United States, 1980–2012. *JAMA* 2014;312:1218–1226

7. Gregg EW, Li Y, Wang J, et al. Changes in diabetes-related complications in the United States, 1990–2010. *N Engl J Med* 2014;370:1514–1523
8. Hu F. Globalization of diabetes: the role of diet, lifestyle, and genes. *Diabetes Care* 2011;34:1249–1257
9. Egede LE, Dagogo-Jack S. Epidemiology of type 2 diabetes: focus on ethnic minorities. *Med Clin N Am* 2005;89:949–975
10. Dagogo-Jack S. Chapter 3-Complications of Diabetes Mellitus, in Section 9, Metabolism. In: ACP Medicine, A Publication of the American College of Physicians, Nabel EG (Editor-in-Chief), B C Decker, Inc., Philadelphia, 2010. Accessed 16 December 2015
11. UK Prospective Diabetes Study Group. UK Prospective Diabetes Study VIII: study design, progress and performance. *Diabetologia* 1991;34: 877–890
12. Spijkerman AM, Dekker JM, Nijpels G, et al. Microvascular complications at time of diagnosis of type 2 diabetes are similar among diabetic patients detected by targeted screening and patients newly diagnosed in general practice: the Hoorn screening study. *Diabetes Care* 2003;26: 2604–2608
13. American Diabetes Association. Economic costs of diabetes in the U.S. in 2017. *Diabetes Care* 2018;41:917–928
14. American Diabetes Association. Economic costs of diabetes in the U.S. in 2012. *Diabetes Care* 2013;36:1033–1046
15. Kaufman FR. Type 2 diabetes mellitus in children and youth: a new epidemic. *J Pediatr Endocrinol Metab* 2002;15(Suppl. 2):737–744
16. Olmos P, A'Hern R, Heaton DA, et al. The significance of the concordance rate for type 1 (insulin-dependent) diabetes in identical twins. *Diabetologia* 1988;31:747–750
17. Granner DK, O'Brien RM. Molecular physiology and genetics of NIDDM. *Diabetes Care* 1992;15:369–388
18. Willemsen G, Ward KJ, Bell CG, et al. The concordance and heritability of type 2 diabetes in 34,166 twin pairs from international twin registers: the Discordant Twin (DISCOTWIN) Consortium. *Twin Res Hum Genet* 2015;18:762–771
19. Weyer C, Bogardus C, Mott DM, Pratley R. The natural history of insulin secretory dysfunction and insulin resistance in the pathogenesis of type 2 diabetes mellitus. *J Clin Invest* 1999;104:787–794
20. Rieck S, Kaestner KH. Expansion of beta-cell mass in response to pregnancy. *Trends Endocrinol Metab* 2010;21:151–158
21. Dagogo-Jack S, Santiago JV. Pathophysiology of type 2 diabetes and modes of action of therapeutic interventions. *Arch Intern Med* 1997;157: 1802–1817

22. DeFronzo RA. Insulin resistance, lipotoxicity, type 2 diabetes and atherosclerosis: the missing links. The Claude Bernard Lecture 2009. *Diabetologia* 2010;53:1270–1287
23. Cepeda M, Muka T, Ikram MA, Franco OH, Schoufour JD. Seasonality of insulin resistance, glucose, and insulin among middle-aged and elderly population: the Rotterdam Study. *J Clin Endocrinol Metab* 2018;103: 946–955
24. Eaton S. Control of mitochondrial beta-oxidation flux. *Prog Lipid Res* 2002;41:197–239
25. Lu H, Bogdanovic E, Yu Z, et al. Combined hyperglycemia- and hyperinsulinemia-induced insulin resistance in adipocytes is associated with dual signaling defects mediated by PKC-ζ. *Endocrinology* 2018;159:1658–1677
26. Ruderman NB, Saha AK, Vavvas D, Witters LA. Malonyl-CoA, fuel sensing, and insulin resistance. *Am J Physiol* 1999;276:E1–E18
27. Rasmussen BB, Holmbäck UC, Volpi E, et al. Malonyl coenzyme A and the regulation of functional carnitine palmitoyltransferase-1 activity and fat oxidation in human skeletal muscle. *J Clin Invest* 2002;110:1687–1693
28. Defronzo RA. Banting Lecture. From the triumvirate to the ominous octet: a new paradigm for the treatment of type 2 diabetes mellitus. *Diabetes* 2009;58:773–795
29. Solinas G, Borén J, Dulloo AG. De novo lipogenesis in metabolic homeostasis: more friend than foe? *Mol Metab* 2015;4:367–377
30. Larson-Meyer DE, Heilbronn LK, Redman LM, et al. Effect of calorie restriction with or without exercise on insulin sensitivity, β-cell function, fat cell size, and ectopic lipid in overweight subjects. *Diabetes Care* 2006;29:1337–1344
31. Kelley DE. Effects of weight loss on glucose homeostasis in NIDDM. *Diabetes Rev* 1995;3:366–377
32. Rogers MA, Yamamoto C, King DS, et al. Improvement in glucose tolerance after one week of exercise in patients with mild NIDDM. *Diabetes Care* 1988;11:613–618
33. Mikines KJ, Sonne B, Farrell PA, et al. Effect of physical exercise on sensitivity and responsiveness to insulin in humans. *Am J Physiol* 1988;254:E248–E259
34. Goodyear LJ, Kahn BB. Exercise, glucose transport, and insulin sensitivity. *Annu Rev Med* 1988;49:235–261
35. Ehm MG, Karnoub MC, Sakul H, et al.; American Diabetes Association GENNID Study Group. Genetics of NIDDM: genome wide search for type 2 diabetes susceptibility genes in four American populations. *Am J Hum Genet* 2000;66:1871–1881

36. McCarthy M, Zeggini E. Genome-wide association studies in type 2 diabetes. *Curr Diab Rep* 2009;9:164–171
37. Hivert MF, Jablonski KA, Perreault L, et al. Updated genetic score based on 34 confirmed type 2 diabetes loci is associated with diabetes incidence and regression to normoglycemia in the Diabetes Prevention Program. *Diabetes* 2011;60:1340–1348
38. Dagogo-Jack S. Predicting diabetes: our relentless quest for genomic nuggets. *Diabetes Care* 2012;35:193–195
39. Fujimoto WY, Leonetti DL, Kinyoun JL, et al. Prevalence of diabetes mellitus and impaired glucose tolerance among second-generation Japanese-American men. *Diabetes* 1987;36:721–729
40. Li W, Dorans KS, Wilker EH, et al. Ambient air pollution, adipokines, and glucose homeostasis: The Framingham Heart Study. *Environ Int* 2018;111:14–22
41. Xu X, Yavar Z, Verdin M, et al. Effect of early particulate air pollution exposure on obesity in mice: role of p47phox. *Arterioscler Thromb Vasc Biol* 2010;30:2518–2527
42. Debelea D, Hanson RL, Lindsay RS, et al. Intrauterine exposure to diabetes conveys risks for type 2 diabetes and obesity: a study of discordant sibships. *Diabetes* 1999;49:2208–2211
43. Pettitt DJ, Aleck KA, Baird HR, et al. Congenital susceptibility to NIDDM: role of intrauterine environment. *Diabetes* 1988;37:622–628
44. Fernandez-Twinn DS, Hjort L, Novakovic B, et al. Intrauterine programming of obesity and type 2 diabetes. *Diabetologia* 2019;62:1789–1801
45. Dagogo-Jack S. *Diabetes Risks from Prescription and Nonprescription Drugs: Mechanisms and Approaches to Risk Reduction*. Alexandria, VA, American Diabetes Association, 2016
46. Dagogo-Jack S, Ed. *Diabetes Mellitus in Developing Countries and Underserved Communities.* 1st ed. New York, Springer, 2017
47. Shan Z, Ma H, Xie M, et al. Sleep duration and risk of type 2 diabetes: a meta-analysis of prospective studies. *Diabetes Care* 2015;38:529–537

Chapter 2

Prediabetes: Evolution of Terminology, Global Estimates, and Diagnosis

Prediabetes

The term "prediabetes" has been used in the medical literature since 1918.[1] The term first appeared in the title of a *Diabetes* article in 1953.[2] For lay readers, prediabetes was first introduced in the 1934 *Oxford English Dictionary* and was defined as "preclinical or early diabetes mellitus, especially as detected by a slightly elevated blood glucose level or impaired glucose tolerance." More recently, prediabetes was reintroduced at a joint press conference by the U.S. Department of Health and Human Services (HHS) and the American Diabetes Association (ADA) on 27 March 2002 during the announcement of the key findings of the Diabetes Prevention Program: "HHS and the ADA are using the new term 'prediabetes' to describe an increasingly common condition in which blood glucose levels are higher than normal but not yet diabetic—known in medicine as impaired glucose tolerance or impaired fasting glucose. Studies have shown that most people with this condition go on to develop type 2 diabetes within 10 years."[3] The Centers for Disease Control and Prevention estimates that 88 million U.S. adults aged 18 years or older (34.5% of the adult U.S. population) had prediabetes in 2018.[4] Worldwide, more than 374 million adults have prediabetes.[5]

As an intermediate stage between normal glucose regulation (i.e., normal fasting plasma glucose and normal 2-h plasma glucose [2hPG]) and type 2 diabetes, prediabetes is currently defined by the presence of impaired fasting glucose and/or impaired glucose tolerance.[6] The impaired fasting glucose criterion for prediabetes is met if the fasting plasma glucose level is between 100 and 125 mg/dL (5.5 and 6.9 mmol/L), and the impaired glucose tolerance criterion is met if the 2hPG level is between 140 and 199 mg/dL (7.8 and 11.0 mmol/L) during a standard 75-g oral glucose tolerance test[6] (Fig. 2.1). In 2009, an international expert committee recommended that the HbA_{1c} (A1C) test be added as one of the criteria for diagnoses of diabetes and prediabetes, initially setting the cutoffs for prediabetes at 6.0 to <6.5% (42–48 mmol/mol).[7] The 2010 ADA Clinical Practice Recommendations

	Normal	Prediabetes	Diabetes
Fasting Glucose	FPG <100 mg/dL (<5.5 mmol/L)	FPG 100–125 mg/dL (5.5–6.9 mmol/L)	FPG ≥126 mg/dL (≥7.0 mmol/L)
Oral Glucose Tolerance Test	2hPG <140 mg/dL (<7.8 mmol/L)	2hPG 140–199 mg/dL (7.8–11.0 mmol/L)	2hPG ≥200 mg/dL (≥11.0 mmol/L)
HbA_{1c}	HbA_{1c} <5.7% (<39 mmol/mol)	HbA_{1c} 5.7–6.4% (39–46 mmol/mol)	HbA_{1c} >6.5% (>46 mmol/mol)

Figure 2.1—Criteria for the diagnosis of diabetes and prediabetes.[8]

adopted the new A1C criterion for diagnosing prediabetes but amended the cut-offs to 5.7–6.4% (39–46 mmol/mol),[8] which has been in effect since then. Before these recommendations, the diagnosis of diabetes and prediabetes was based solely on measurement of fasting plasma glucose levels or the standard 75-g oral glucose tolerance test.[9,10]

With the 2010 ADA recommendation, the diagnosis of prediabetes can now be made using fasting plasma glucose, 2hPG, or A1C values (Fig. 2.1). The convenience (no requirement for fasting), higher analytical stability, and prognostic value regarding prediction of microvascular complications are real advantages of using the A1C test for diagnosis of diabetes. However, caution is required when using A1C for diagnosis of prediabetes because of the numerous factors that could affect the presumed correlation between average blood glucose and $A1C_c$ values in certain situations.[11] The latter include hemolytic anemia, iron deficiency, hemoglobinopathies, pregnancy, and uremia, among others.[11] Thus, it is prudent to confirm marginal results with actual blood glucose measurement for the diagnosis of prediabetes.[11]

Impaired Glucose Tolerance and Impaired Fasting Glucose

The two glucose-based definitions of prediabetes—impaired glucose tolerance and impaired fasting glucose—have different origins and metabolic connotations, and identify different populations. The definition of impaired glucose tolerance was originally proposed by the World Health Organization and has been in use for decades.[12,13] That definition includes a normal fasting plasma glucose level and a 2hPG value that lies between 140 and 199 mg/dL during a standard 75-g oral glucose tolerance test.[12,13] As a dynamic test, the oral glucose tolerance test probes the integrity of glucoregulatory responses when stressed with a challenge stimulus of an oral glucose load. The critical glucoregulatory responses to such a challenge, aimed at restoring glucose homeostasis and dampening blood glucose excursions, require prompt secretion of insulin by the pancreatic islet β-cells and intact insulin action (sensitivity) at target sites, principally skeletal muscle and adipose tissue. Thus, the inability to return blood glucose to a healthy level, 2 h after the oral glucose load, signifies glucose intolerance due to impairments in the glucoregulatory processes. Consonant with this premise, numerous studies have established impaired glucose tolerance as a prediabetic state that is associated with insulin resistance and impaired insulin secretion.[6,14–17]

In contrast, the term "impaired fasting glucose" was first introduced by the ADA in 1997 and defined as a fasting plasma glucose value between 110 and 125 mg/dL.[9] In September 2003, the ADA revised the definition of normal fasting glucose (NFG) as <100 mg/dL,[18] thereby redefining impaired fasting glucose as any fasting plasma glucose value between 100 and 125 mg/dL. These definitions and re-definitions of NFG and impaired fasting glucose seemingly occurred without a precise physiological or pathophysiological understanding of the gradations in metabolic, glucoregulatory, or cardiovascular risks across fasting plasma glucose thresholds within the nondiabetic range.[19] The requirement for an overnight fast (lasting ~8–12 h) means that the fasting plasma glucose test is a measure of endogenous glucose production, in contrast to the 2hPG test, which is a measure of glucose disposal. The key contributors to endogenous glucose production include hepatic glycolysis and gluconeogenesis, lipolysis (with release of gluconeogenic precursors), and proteolysis (with outflow of gluconeogenic amino acids from the muscle bed). Because all of these processes are inhibited by insulin, an elevated fasting plasma glucose can be explained by inadequate overnight basal insulin secretion and/or impaired insulin action at the hepatocyte, adipocyte, and myocyte levels. Indeed, significant defects in insulin action and secretion are consistently demonstrable in people with impaired fasting glucose.[15,16,20–23]

Insulin Resistance in Prediabetes

Our group tested the hypothesis that variations in fasting plasma glucose levels within the normal range reflect differences in insulin sensitivity and β-cell function.[23] Using results of the 75-g oral glucose tolerance test, we classified study participants (mean age [± SD] 36.4 ± 1.7 years; BMI 20–56 kg/m^2) as having NFG (<100 mg/dL) or impaired fasting glucose (fasting plasma glucose 100–125 mg/dL). The NFG group was subdivided into low-NFG (<90 mg/dL) and high-NFG (90–99 mg/dL). Using the 2-h oral glucose tolerance test plasma glucose value, we further classified participants as having normal glucose tolerance or impaired glucose tolerance. Insulin resistance was calculated using homeostasis model assessment–insulin resistance (HOMA-IR),[24] and insulin sensitivity was measured directly using the hyperinsulinemic-euglycemic clamp (ISI-clamp).[25] β-Cell function was assessed by calculating the insulinogenic index, homeostasis model assessment of β-cell function (HOMA-B), and oral disposition index.[24,26] Individuals with low-NFG had the best glucoregulatory profile compared with the other groups: lowest glucose and insulin excursions and glucose area under the curve during oral glucose tolerance test, lowest insulin resistance, and highest disposition index. There was a gradation of impairment in glucose tolerance, insulin sensitivity, and disposition index across the spectrum from high-NFG, through impaired fasting glucose to combined impaired fasting glucose plus impaired glucose tolerance status.[23]

Clamp-derived insulin sensitivity (Insulin Sensitivity Index-clamp) was similar among low-NFG and high-NFG subjects (0.109 ± 0.011 vs. 0.117 ± 0.015) but significantly lower by ~20% in subjects with impaired fasting glucose (0.088 ± 0.009, $P = 0.04$) and by ~80% among subjects with combined impaired fasting glucose plus impaired glucose tolerance (0.022 ± 0.003) ($P = 0.0014$ vs. low-NFG, 0.0027 vs. high-NFG, and 0.0011 vs. isolated impaired fasting glucose) (Fig. 2.2). Interestingly,

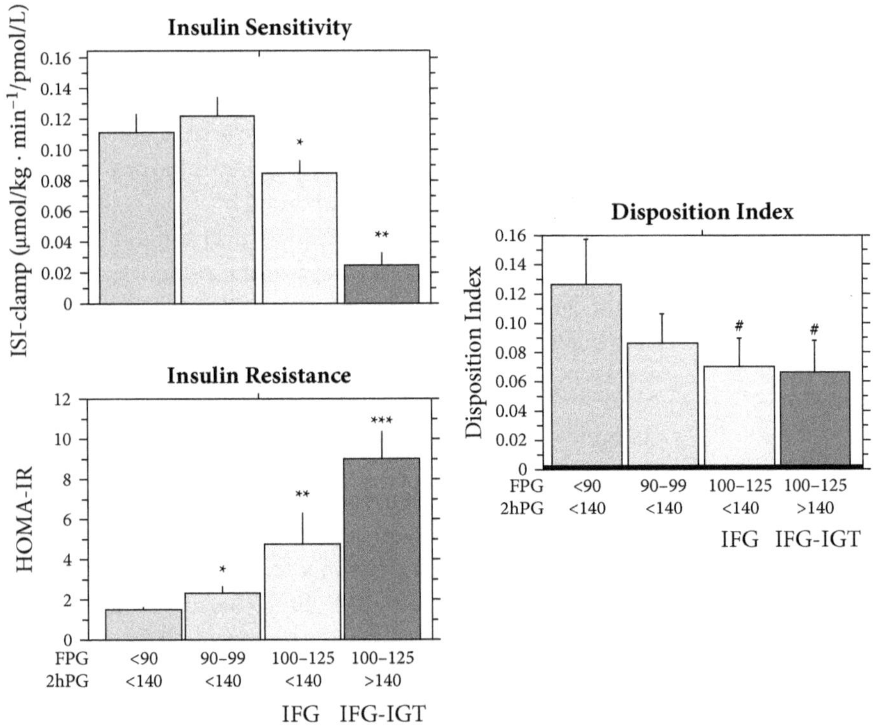

Figure 2.2—Insulin sensitivity and insulin secretion (disposition index) subjects with low-NGT, high-NGT, or impaired fasting glucose with or without impaired glucose tolerance.[23] $^{*}P = 0.04$; $^{**}P = 0.002$; $^{***}P < 0.0001$; $\#P = 0.02$.

estimates of insulin action calculated from HOMA-IR significantly differentiated subjects with low-NFG from those with high-NFG by showing a two-fold increase in insulin resistance among the latter. The HOMA-IR data also showed a four-fold and an eight-fold increase in insulin resistance in subjects with impaired fasting glucose and combined impaired fasting glucose plus impaired glucose tolerance, respectively, compared with the low-NFG group. In contrast, the ISI-clamp data showed only a 20% decrease in impaired fasting glucose versus low-NFG and an 80% decrease in combined impaired fasting glucose plus impaired glucose tolerance versus low-NFG in whole-body (predominantly skeletal muscle) insulin sensitivity.[23]

The reasons for the discrepancy in the magnitudes of difference in insulin action estimated by the two methods might relate to the metabolic targets being measured. As a derivative of fasting glucose and insulin values, HOMA-IR assesses mostly hepatic insulin resistance; the hyperinsulinemic-euglycemic clamp method measures whole-body (predominantly skeletal muscle) glucose disposal. Thus, the metabolic data obtained by the two methods are related but not necessarily identical. The HOMA-IR data suggest that the high-NFG subjects had significant hepatic insulin resistance compared with subjects with low-NFG. In contrast, the euglycemic clamp data indicate that skeletal muscle glucose uptake under conditions of exogenous hyperinsulinemia might be similar between low-NFG and high-NFG groups. Compared with the normoglycemic groups, subjects with impaired fasting glucose and those with combined impaired fasting glucose plus impaired glucose tolerance were significantly insulin resistant by both the clamp and HOMA-IR methods; however, the HOMA-IR data suggest that hepatic insulin resistance is an early defect in people with impaired fasting glucose, with superimposed impaired whole-body glucose disposal (as measured with clamp) in people with impaired glucose tolerance. This notion is supported by a study of Mexican American offspring of parents with type 2 diabetes in which insulin-stimulated glucose disposal was similar in subjects with normal glucose tolerance and impaired fasting glucose, but was reduced by 42% in subjects with impaired glucose tolerance and by 48% in those with combined impaired fasting glucose plus impaired glucose tolerance.[17]

Insulin Secretion in Prediabetes

The insulin secretion data across the four comparison groups were quite interesting. Among normoglycemic subjects, basal (fasting) plasma insulin levels were similar between the low-NFG and high-NFG groups. When compared to normoglycemic subjects, fasting plasma insulin levels were higher among subjects with impaired fasting glucose and combined impaired fasting glucose plus impaired glucose tolerance (Table 2.1). Estimates of β-cell function derived from both the

Table 2.1—Indices of Insulin Action and Secretion in Subjects With Low-NFG, High-NFG, or Impaired Fasting Glucose With or Without Impaired Glucose Tolerance[23]

	Low-NFG	High-NFG	Isolated IFG	IFG + IGT	*P*
GDR (μmol/kg · min)	34.6 ± 4.00	37.9 ± 4.82	29.1 ± 3.56	13.3 ± 1.41	0.0009
Steady-state clamp plasma insulin (μU/mL)	66.9 ± 9.30	66.7 ± 6.28	60.4 ± 9.45	79.1 ± 10.1	0.013
ISI-clamp (μmol/kg · min/pmol/L)	0.109 ± 0.011	0.117 ± 0.015	0.088 ± 0.009	0.022 ± 0.003	0.0011
HOMA-IR	1.43 ± 0.11	2.30 ± 0.36	4.78 ± 1.26	9.00 ± 1.41	<0.0001
Glucose AUC (mg · dL^{-1} · min^{-1})	7,036 ± 1,075	9,722 ± 1,202	13,578 ± 1,543	18,176 ± 2,102	0.0035
Fasting insulin (μU/mL)	7.0 ± 0.60	9.9 ± 1.5	17.3 ± 4.10	30.6 ± 5.5	<0.0001
Insulinogenic index	1.20 ± 0.32	1.03 ± 0.21	1.18 ± 0.51	2.50 ± 0.58	0.05
HOMA-B (%)	143 ± 29.9	114 ± 18.4	131 ± 24.8	222 ± 31.5	0.048

GDR, glucose disposal rate at steady-state during hyperinsulinemic-euglycemic clamp; glucose AUC, area under the glucose curve during a standard 75-g oral glucose tolerance curve; HOMA-IR, homeostasis model of insulin resistance.

HOMA-B and insulinogenic index indicated no significant differences in insulin secretion among subjects with low-NFG, high-NFG, or isolated impaired fasting glucose (Table 2.1). However, the subjects with combined impaired fasting glucose plus impaired glucose tolerance had values for HOMA-B and insulinogenic index that were higher than values for subjects in the other groups.

Because insulin secretion is best assessed in relation to ambient insulin sensitivity, the disposition index (the product of acute insulin secretory response to glucose and insulin sensitivity index) was analyzed. Compared to low-NFG subjects, the disposition index was lower by 32.8% in high-NFG subjects, by 45.6% in subjects with isolated impaired fasting glucose, and by 49.8% ($P < 0.02$) in subjects with combined impaired fasting glucose plus impaired glucose tolerance (Fig. 2.1).[23] Thus, prediabetes is associated with impaired insulin secretion when corrected for ambient insulin resistance.

Clearly, insulin resistance and pancreatic β-cell dysfunction, well-known defects in type 2 diabetes, are demonstrable in individuals with prevalent prediabetes (impaired fasting glucose and impaired glucose tolerance) as well.[5] Adiposity (as measured by BMI) correlated directly with fasting insulin and inversely with insulin sensitivity, which justifies the well-known practice of using fasting insulin as a surrogate for insulin sensitivity (Fig. 2.3*A*, *C*, and *D*). Insulin sensitivity was inversely correlated with glycemia, even within the NFG range, with increases in fasting plasma glucose levels from 70 to 125 mg/dL being associated with a greater than three-fold decline in insulin sensitivity (Fig. 2.3).[23] Studies in adolescents[15,20,26] and adults[16,17,22] are concordant in showing the presence of a β-cell defect in subjects with isolated impaired fasting glucose or impaired glucose tolerance, and severe insulin resistance in those with combined impaired fasting glucose plus impaired glucose tolerance.

Focusing on early glucose abnormalities (including high-NFG, impaired fasting glucose, and impaired glucose tolerance) is justified by the link between mild dysglycemia and increased cardiometabolic risk.[16,27–31] Individuals with fasting plasma glucose <90 mg/dL are generally more insulin sensitive than individuals with fasting plasma glucose between 90 and 99 mg/dL, with the latter being more likely to progress to prediabetes,[23,32] with subsequent risks of developing type 2 diabetes and vascular complications.[33,34] Thus, fasting glycemia in the 90–99 mg/dL range (the pre-impaired fasting glucose or "pre-prediabetes" stage) appears to connote incipient transition to a higher-risk cardiometabolic risk phenotype.[23]

Interestingly, when prediabetes is defined solely by A1C values of 5.7–6.4%, no clear separation of insulin sensitivity or insulin secretion can be discerned between normal and "prediabetes" subjects.[35] Ebenibo et al.[35] studied 280 nondiabetic adults (mean age 44.2 ± 10.6 years). After clinical assessment, each study participant underwent a standard 75-g oral glucose tolerance test and measurement of A1C level. Participants were then scheduled for two additional outpatient visits

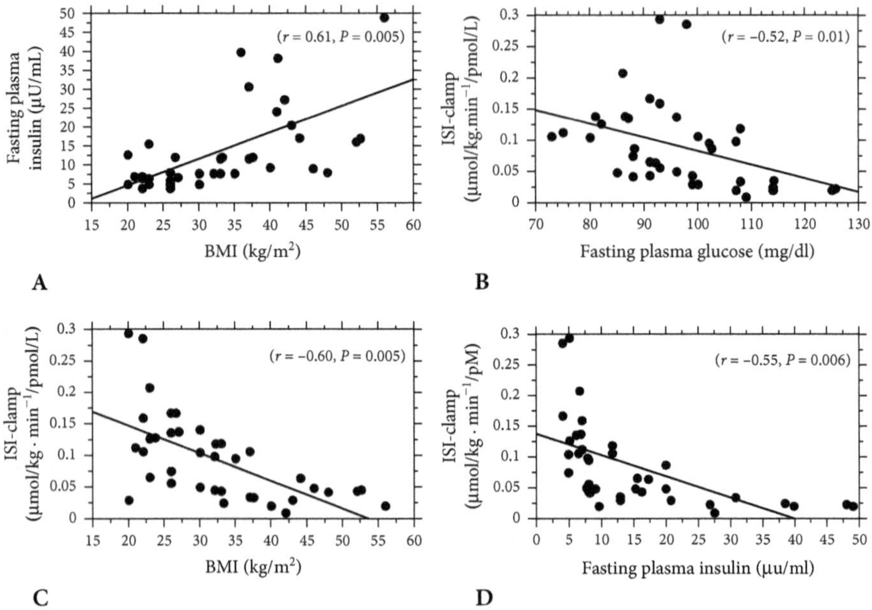

Figure 2.3—Correlations of fasting plasma insulin with BMI (*A*) and of insulin sensitivity (ISI-clamp) with fasting plasma glucose (*B*), BMI (*C*), and fasting plasma insulin (*D*) in subjects with low-NGT, high-NGT, or impaired fasting glucose with or without impaired glucose tolerance.[23]

during which insulin sensitivity (hyperinsulinemic-euglycemic clamp) and acute insulin secretion (frequently sampled intravenous glucose tolerance test) were measured. The disposition index (insulin secretion adjusted for ambient insulin sensitivity) was also recorded. Based on the A1C level, participants were classified as having prediabetes (A1C 5.7–6.4%) or as normal (A1C <5.7%), according to the ADA criteria.[35] When the two groups were matched for age and BMI, individuals with A1C-defined "prediabetes" were indistinguishable from those whose A1C was <5.7% in terms of insulin sensitivity, insulin secretion, or disposition index, due to considerable overlap.[35]

Clearly, unlike glucose-defined prediabetes (impaired fasting glucose or impaired glucose tolerance) status, an A1C range of 5.7–6.4% does not reliably identify individuals with impaired insulin action or secretion, the classic defects underlying the pathophysiology of prediabetes.[35] If used as a screening test for convenience, **clinicians should confirm A1C values in the prediabetes range with blood glucose measurement.** Furthermore, a comprehensive assessment with an oral glucose tolerance test that simultaneously documents and classifies the prediabetes states of impaired fasting glucose, impaired glucose tolerance, or combined impaired fasting glucose plus impaired glucose tolerance would help separate out the potentially higher-risk subgroup with combined impaired fasting glucose plus impaired glucose tolerance and guide therapeutic decision-making.[36–38]

References

1. Auer J, Kleiner IS. Morphine hyperglycemia in dogs with experimental pancreatic deficiency. *J Exp Med* 1918;27:49–63
2. MCullagh EP. A pre-diabetic state in parents of overweight babies. *Diabetes* 1953;2:160–161
3. U.S. Department of Health and Human Services, American Diabetes Association. Press release. 27 March 2002. Washington, DC, U.S. Department of Health and Human Services, 2002. Available from http://wayback.archiveit.org/3926/20130930184836/http://archive.hhs.gov/news/press/2002pres/20020327.htm. Accessed 17 August 2018
4. Centers for Disease Control and Prevention. *National Diabetes Statistics Report, 2020. Estimates of Diabetes and Its Burden in the United States.* Atlanta, GA, Centers for Disease Control and Prevention, U.S. Department of Health and Human Services. Available from https://www.cdc.gov/diabetes/pdfs/data/statistics/national-diabetes-statistics-report.pdf. Accessed 28 October 2020
5. International Diabetes Federation. *IDF Diabetes Atlas.* 9th ed. Brussels, Belgium, International Diabetes Federation, 2019
6. American Diabetes Association. *Standards of Medical Care in Diabetes—2021.* Diagnosis and Classification of Diabetes Mellitus. *Diabetes Care* 2021;44:S1–S232
7. International Expert Committee. International Expert Committee Report on the Role of the A1C Assay in the Diagnosis of Diabetes. *Diabetes Care* 2009;32:1327–1334
8. American Diabetes Association. Diagnosis and classification of diabetes mellitus. *Diabetes Care* 2010;33(Suppl. 1):S62–S69
9. Expert Committee on the Diagnosis and Classification of Diabetes Mellitus. Report of the Expert Committee on the Diagnosis and Classification of Diabetes Mellitus. *Diabetes Care* 1997;20:1183–1197
10. World Health Organization. *Definition, Diagnosis and Classification of Diabetes Mellitus and Its Complications: Report of a WHO Consultation. Part 1. Diagnosis and Classification of Diabetes Mellitus.* Geneva, World Health Org., 1999, pp. 1–59
11. Dagogo-Jack S. Pitfalls in the use of HbA_{1c} as a diagnostic test: the ethnic conundrum. *Nat Rev Endocrinol* 2010;6:589–593

12. World Health Organization. *Diabetes Mellitus: Report of a WHO Study Group.* Geneva, World Health Org., 1985 (Tech. Rep. Ser., no. 727)
13. World Health Organization (WHO/IDF) Consultation. *Definition and Diagnosis of Diabetes Mellitus and Intermediate Hyperglycemia.* Geneva, World Health Org., 2006. Available from http://www.who.int/diabetes/publications/Definition%20and%20diagnosis%20of%20diabetes_new.pdf. Accessed 30 January 2020
14. Haffner SM, Miettinen H, Gaskill SP, Stern MP. Decreased insulin action and insulin secretion predict the development of impaired glucose tolerance. *Diabetologia* 1996;39:1201–1207
15. Bacha F, Gungor N, Lee S, Arslanian SA. In vivo insulin sensitivity and secretion in obese youth: what are the differences between NGT, impaired glucose tolerance and type 2 diabetes? *Diabetes Care* 2009;32:100–105
16. Novoa FJ, Boronat M, Saavedra P, et al. Differences in cardiovascular risk factors, insulin resistance, and insulin secretion in individuals with normal glucose tolerance and in subjects with impaired glucose regulation: the Telde Study. *Diabetes Care* 2005;28:2388–2393
17. Abdul-Ghani MA, Jenkinson CP, Richardson DK, et al. Insulin secretion and action in subjects with impaired fasting glucose and impaired glucose tolerance. *Diabetes* 2006;55:1430–1435
18. Genuth S, Alberti KG, Bennett P, et al.; Expert Committee on the Diagnosis and Classification of Diabetes Mellitus. Follow-up report on the diagnosis of diabetes mellitus. *Diabetes Care* 2003;26:3160–3167
19. Schriger DL, Lorber B. Lowering the cut point for impaired fasting glucose: where is the evidence? Where is the logic? *Diabetes Care* 2004;27:592–601
20. Cali' AM, Bonadonna RC, Trombetta M, et al. Metabolic abnormalities underlying the different prediabetic phenotypes in obese adolescents. *J Clin Endocrinol Metab* 2008;93:1767–1773
21. Faerch K, Vaag A, Holst JJ, et al. Impaired fasting glycaemia vs impaired glucose tolerance: similar impairment of pancreatic alpha and beta cell function but differential roles of incretin hormones and insulin action. *Diabetologia* 2008;51:853–861
22. Hong J, Gui MH, Gu WQ, et al. Differences in insulin resistance and pancreatic B-cell function in obese subjects with isolated impaired glucose tolerance and isolated impaired fasting glucose. *Diabet Med* 2008;25:73–79

23. Dagogo-Jack S, Askari H, Tykodi G. Glucoregulatory physiology in subjects with low-normal, high-normal, or impaired fasting glucose. *J Clin Endocrinol Metab* 2009;94:2031–2036
24. Matthews D, Hosker J, Rudenski A, et al. Homeostasis model assessment: insulin resistance and beta cell function from fasting plasma glucose and insulin concentrations in man. *Diabetologia* 1985;28:412–419
25. DeFronzo RA, Tobin JD, Andres R. Glucose clamp technique: a method for quantifying insulin secretion and resistance. *Am J Physiol* 1979;237: E214–E223
26. Uwaifo GI, Fallon EM, Chin J, et al. Indices of insulin action, disposal, and secretion derived from fasting samples and clamps in normal glucose-tolerant black and white children. *Diabetes Care* 2002;25:2081–2087
27. Cerasi E, Luft R. The prediabetic state, its nature and consequences: a look toward the future. *Diabetes* 1972;21(Suppl. 2):685–694
28. Eschwege E, Richard JL, Thibult N, et al. Coronary heart disease mortality in relation with diabetes, blood glucose and plasma insulin levels: the Paris Prospective Study, ten years later. *Horm Metab Res Suppl* 1985;15:41–46
29. Khaw KT, Wareham N, Bingham S, et al. Association of hemoglobin A1c with cardiovascular disease and mortality in adults: the European prospective investigation into cancer in Norfolk. *Ann Intern Med* 2004;141:413–420
30. Weir G, Bonner-Weir S. Five stages of evolving progression to diabetes. *Diabetes* 2004;53:S16–S21
31. Dagogo-Jack S, Edeoga C. Understanding and identifying pre-diabetes: can we halt the diabetes epidemic? *European Endocrinology* 2008;4: 16–18
32. Dagogo-Jack S, Edeoga C, Ebenibo S, et al.; Pathobiology of Prediabetes in a Biracial Cohort (POP-ABC) Research Group. Lack of racial disparity in incident prediabetes and glycemic progression among black and white offspring of parents with type 2 diabetes: the Pathobiology of Prediabetes in a Biracial Cohort (POP-ABC) study. *J Clin Endocrinol Metab* 2014;99:E1078–E1087
33. Tabák A, Herder C, Rathmann W, et al. Prediabetes: a high-risk state for diabetes development. *Lancet* 2012;379:2279–2290
34. Brannick B, Wynn A, Dagogo-Jack S. Prediabetes as a toxic environment for the initiation of microvascular and macrovascular complications. *Exp Biol Med (Maywood)* 2016;241:1323–1331
35. Ebenibo S, Edeoga C, Wan J, Dagogo-Jack S. Glucoregulatory function among African Americans and European Americans with normal or pre-diabetic hemoglobin A1c levels. *Metabolism* 2014;63:767–772

36. Nathan DM, Davidson MB, DeFronzo RA, et al. Impaired fasting glucose and impaired glucose tolerance. *Diabetes Care* 2007;30:753–759
37. Pour OR, Dagogo-Jack S. Prediabetes as a therapeutic target. *Clin Chem* 2011;57:215–220
38. Brannick B, Dagogo-Jack S. Prediabetes and cardiovascular disease: pathophysiology and interventions for prevention and risk reduction. *Endocrinol Metab Clin North Am* 2018;47:33–50

Chapter 3

Demographic, Anthropometric, and Behavioral Predictors of Progression from Normal Glucose Regulation to Prediabetes

Transition from Normal Glucose Regulation to Prediabetes

In contrast to the numerous studies on the transition from prediabetes to type 2 diabetes (discussed later), relatively few studies have focused on the transition from normal glucose regulation to prediabetes.[1–8] Among a high-risk population of 254 Pima Indians with baseline normoglycemia, 79 subjects (31%) progressed to prediabetes (impaired glucose tolerance) during a mean follow-up period of 4 years, yielding an annualized prediabetes incidence rate of 9.5%.[1,2] Another study that reported on incident prediabetes was the Baltimore Longitudinal Study of Aging (BLSA), which used biennial oral glucose tolerance tests to document glycemic progression in an adult, predominantly white (96%) population selected from residents of Baltimore, Maryland.[3] Of the 488 BLSA participants with normal glucose tolerance at enrollment, 62% had progressed to prediabetes by 10 years of follow-up, yielding an incident prediabetes rate of 6.2% per year.[3]

Two studies conducted in Asia reported on prevalent[4] and incident[5] rates of prediabetes. In a cross-sectional study of 27,552 Chinese adults (aged ≥20 years), the prevalent rate of prediabetes was reported as 27.2%.[4] The other study enrolled 3,879 Japanese subjects (mean age ~50 years) with normal glucose regulation in a longitudinal study with the prespecified primary outcome of incident prediabetes (defined as combined fasting plasma glucose >110 mg/dL [6.1 mmol/L] and A1C >5.5%).[5] After 5 years of follow-up, the combined prediabetes end points occurred in 21 participants; either of the two prediabetes criteria occurred in another 1,730 subjects, and the remainder (2,128 subjects) did not manifest any glycemic departure from their original normal glucose regulation status.[5] The progression from normal glucose regulation to at least one prediabetes criterion occurred in 45.7% (1,751 of 3,879) of Japanese subjects during 5 years of follow-up, yielding an annualized prediabetes incidence of 9%.[5] The factors significantly associated with increased risk of transition from normal glucose regulation to any prediabetes end point included baseline hematocrit, alanine aminotransferase, triglyceride, and LDL cholesterol levels.[5]

A more diverse population of initially normoglycemic African American and European American offspring of parents with type 2 diabetes were enrolled in the Pathobiology of Prediabetes in a Biracial Cohort (POP-ABC) study.[6–8] POP-ABC study participants were followed with quarterly fasting plasma glucose measurements and annual oral glucose tolerance tests for 5 years. The primary outcome was occurrence of incident prediabetes (impaired fasting glucose and/or impaired glucose tolerance).[6–8] During a total follow-up period of 5.5 years (mean 2.62 years), ~30% of POP-ABC participants developed prediabetes (annualized rate ~11%).[8] The incidence of prediabetes was similar in African American and European American offspring of parents with type 2 diabetes, indicating that parental history of type 2 diabetes probably attenuated any ethnic disparities in early glucose abnormalities.

Taken together, these studies, reported from different continents and conducted in different populations, found a surprisingly narrow range of 6–11% as the observed annual rate of progression from normoglycemia to incident prediabetes.[1–8] Because initial transition to prediabetes is a necessary step toward the development of type 2 diabetes, predicting individuals at risk for such incident dysglycemia would be valuable information for the precise target of any preventive interventions. What follows is a discussion of those factors that have been associated with the risk of progression from normal glucose regulation to prediabetes.

Predictors of Initial Transition to Prediabetes

Demographic predictors

The significant baseline demographic predictors of incident prediabetes include age and sex. In the POP-ABC study, the mean age at baseline of progressors from normal glucose regulation to prediabetes was significantly higher than the age of participants who maintained normoglycemic status during longitudinal follow-up (47 ± 8.9 vs. 43.9 ± 10.7 years, $P = 0.0017$).[8] Additionally, the ratio of people aged 18 to <40 years to people aged 40–65 years was 0.26 among progressors and 0.58 among nonprogressors.[8] Thus, for every participant aged <40 years who progressed to prediabetes, there were 3.8 participants aged 40–65 years who also progressed. Older subjects were more likely to develop incident prediabetes and less likely to maintain normal glucose regulation status during 5.5 years of follow-up[8] (Fig. 3.1).

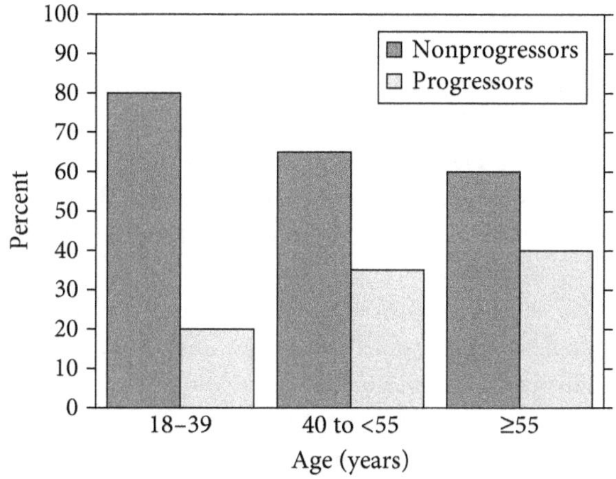

Figure 3.1—Percentage of participants from different age-groups who progressed from normoglycemia to prediabetes (progressors) or maintained normoglycemia (nonprogressors) during 5.5 years of follow-up in the POP-ABC study.[8] *ANOVA $P = 0.0017$.

In the Pima Indian study, the group that experienced glycemic progression had significantly more women than men[2]; in contrast, there were disproportionately more men than women among progressors to incident prediabetes in the POP-ABC study.[8] The male-to-female ratio among progressors was 0.71, compared with 0.29 among nonprogressors.[8] The observation of male preponderance in incident prediabetes among the African Americans and European Americans enrolled in the POP-ABC study is consistent with data from the U.S. National Health and Nutrition Examination Survey (NHANES) 1999–2002[9] and NHANES 2005–2006.[10,11] Both surveys reported a higher prevalence of prediabetes in men than women in cross-sectional national samples representative of the general U.S. population. The reasons for the apparent reversal (more female than male glycemic progressors) in the Pima Indian study are unclear.[2] Notably, despite findings of male preponderance at the prediabetes stage, there is no major sex difference among people with diabetes. Thus, whatever mechanisms that account for sex imbalance during transition from normal glucose regulation to prediabetes are overcome by other mechanisms that restore equilibration between the sexes during subsequent transition from prediabetes to type 2 diabetes.[12]

In the Framingham Offspring Cohort study, individuals with a maternal history of diabetes were more likely to develop prediabetes than individuals with paternal diabetes, although the subsequent risk of type 2 diabetes was similar, regardless of parental sex.[13] In the POP-ABC study, African American offspring were more likely to report maternal diabetes, and European American offspring were more likely to report paternal diabetes, yet there was no racial difference in incident prediabetes or any discernible effect of parental sex on the observed incidence of prediabetes overall.[8] At the molecular level, a variant close to the insulin receptor substrate 1 (*IRS1*) gene (C allele of rs2943641) is associated with insulin resistance and increased type 2 diabetes risk.[14] However, that risk is differentially expressed, based on whether the allele is inherited from the father (increased risk) or the mother (decreased risk).[14]

National cross-sectional surveys in the United States often report a higher prevalence of diagnosed diabetes in African Americans and other ethnic groups compared with European Americans.[9–11,15] However, when individuals with prediabetes from the different ethnic groups were followed for progression to type 2 diabetes, there were no significant differences between European Americans and other ethnic groups in the incidence of type 2 diabetes.[16] Thus, ethnic/racial factors do not seem to play a leading role in predicting progression to type 2 diabetes among individuals who already have developed prediabetes. Theoretically, if African Americans progressed from normal glucose regulation to prediabetes at a higher rate than European Americans, and both groups then developed type 2 diabetes at a similar rate, an initial enrichment of the prediabetes risk pool with African Americans might explain subsequent cross-sectional findings of ethnic disparities in diabetes prevalence. That notion was tested in the POP-ABC study, the findings of which were not supportive. Initially, normoglycemic African Americans and European Americans progressed to prediabetes at a similar rate of ~11% per year.[8]

Much of the racial/ethnic information on prevalent diabetes in the United States was derived from cross-sectional surveys of samples drawn from the U.S. population. Such surveys relied on self-report during telephone interviews. In the 2005–2006 NHANES, 516 people admitted prior communication from a health care professional that they had diabetes (classified as "diagnosed diabetes"); 3,107 people who did not report prior diagnosis of diabetes were tested with blood glucose measurements, the results of which provided an estimate of undiagnosed diabetes and prediabetes.[10] The prevalence of "diagnosed diabetes" (based on self-report) was 12.8% in African Americans and 6.6% in European Americans.[10] Remarkably, the measured blood glucose data from NHANES 2005–2006 showed no significant racial/ethnic differences in the prevalence of undiagnosed diabetes or prediabetes.[10]

The 2011 National Diabetes Fact Sheet estimates for "diagnosed and undiagnosed diabetes" among U.S. adults were 10.2% in European Americans and 18.7% in African Americans.[17] The race/ethnicity-specific estimates for diagnosed diabetes relied on self-reported data from the 2007–2009 National Health Interview Survey.[18] To estimate the prevalence of undiagnosed diabetes and prediabetes, the 2011 National Diabetes Fact Sheet relied on actual blood glucose and A1C measurements.[17] Using these "hard" measures, again, there was no racial/ethnic difference in the prevalence of undiagnosed diabetes or prediabetes.[17] Indeed, none of the national surveys based on blood glucose measurements has indicated a higher prevalence of undiagnosed diabetes or prediabetes in African Americans compared with European Americans.[9–11,19,20] The POP-ABC study findings, thus, are consistent with national cross-sectional data obtained from measured blood glucose values, although they do raise some questions regarding the estimates based on self-reported data that are used for calculating the prevalence of diagnosed diabetes across the various demographic groups.

Anthropometric predictors

The factors that were significantly associated with the risk of escape from normal glucose regulation and development of prediabetes in studies conducted among Pima Indians included weight gain, insulin resistance, and impaired insulin secretion.[2] Significant increases in endogenous (hepatic) glucose production, measured by isotope dilution technique, were not evident during transition from normal glucose tolerance to impaired glucose tolerance, but occurred relatively late during further glycemic progression from impaired glucose tolerance to diabetes.[2] The Pima Indians with persistent normoglycemia during follow-up had a mean weight change of +2.6 kg (~0.65 kg/year) versus +5.6 kg (~1.5 kg/year) in subjects who became dysglycemic and progressed to impaired glucose tolerance.[2] Thus, a weight gain of <1.0 kg/year was protective, whereas a weight gain of >1.0 kg/year was predictive, of early glucose dysregulation among the Pima Indians.[2] Increases in fat mass as well as fat-free mass accounted for the higher weight gain in progressors to prediabetes compared with nonprogressors; however, changes in percent body fat and waist-to-hip ratio reportedly were not different between the comparison groups.[2]

Thus, the absolute amount of weight gain, rather than changes in body composition or fat distribution per se, appeared to predict glycemic progression in the Pima Indian population,[2,21] which is in discord with findings in other populations.[22] Notably, the Pima Indians of Arizona had the highest rate of type 2 diabetes in the world,[23] and some of the mechanistic observations might be unique to that demographic group. The findings from the longitudinal Pima Indian studies support cross-sectional data from a large Chinese study (N = 27,552) that showed significant associations between prevalent prediabetes and adiposity measures, such as BMI and waist circumference. Consistent with the known cardiometabolic risks of visceral adiposity, the Chinese study found that waist circumference had a stronger association with prediabetes than BMI.[4]

In the POP-ABC study, the significant baseline anthropometric variables predictive of incident prediabetes included weight, BMI, waist circumference, total fat mass, and trunk fat mass (Table 3.1).[8,24] POP-ABC participants who developed incident prediabetes had a mean enrollment weight of 90.0 ± 20.4 kg compared to

Table 3.1—Clinical and Biochemical Predictors of Incident Prediabetes among Initially Normoglycemic Adults

Demographic and adiposity measures	Lipids and metabolomic measures
• Older age	• Higher triglycerides
• Male sex	• Higher LDL/lower HDL cholesterol
• Higher BMI	• Higher asparagine/aspartic acid
• Higher waist circumference	• Higher glutamine/glutamic acid
• Higher total body fat mass	• Lower histidine
• Higher abdominal fat mass	• Higher octenoyl carnitine (C8:1)
Glucoregulatory measures	**Behavioral and miscellaneous measures**
• Upper-normal FPG	• Lower physical activity levels
• Upper-normal 2hPG	• Higher blood pressure
• Lower insulin sensitivity	• Lower adiponectin
• Impaired insulin secretion	• Higher hematocrit
• Lower disposition index	• Higher alanine aminotransferase

FPG, fasting plasma glucose; 2hPG, 2-h plasma glucose during oral glucose tolerance test.

82.9 ± 21.7 kg among nonprogressors (*P* = 0.006). During a mean follow-up of 2.62 years, analysis of serial weight measurements showed a mean weight change of 0.63 ± 6.11 kg among nonprogressors compared to 2.54 ± 6.91 kg among progressors (repeated-measures ANOVA *P* = 0.0072).[24] Progressors to prediabetes had a higher baseline waist circumference (99.5 ± 12.5 vs. 90.5 ± 15.3 cm, *P* = 0.002) and showed greater increases in waist circumference during follow-up (1.86 ± 5.80 vs. 1.10 ± 5.44 cm, repeated-measures ANOVA *P* = 0.0001) compared with nonprogressors. Furthermore, POP-ABC study participants who developed incident prediabetes had higher total body fat mass and trunk fat mass at enrollment and showed greater increases in those measures during follow-up, compared with nonprogressors.[24] Thus, in the diverse POP-ABC study population, a weight gain of ~0.2 kg/year was protective, whereas a weight gain of ~1 kg/year was predictive, of glycemic dysregulation, escape from normoglycemia, and developing incident prediabetes.[8]

The relationship between the pattern of weight gain and risk of incident prediabetes observed among POP-ABC study participants (African American and European American offspring of parents with type 2 diabetes) is somewhat akin to that observed in Pima Indians. In both the Pima Indian and POP-ABC study populations, a modest weight gain of ~1–1.5 kg/year was associated with progression from normoglycemia to prediabetes.[2,8] Moreover, the calculated annual incidence rates of prediabetes were comparable in the POP-ABC and Pima Indian study participants (11%/year vs. 9.5%/year).[1,2,8] Although the findings from both studies cannot be compared directly, because of methodological and other reasons, the incidence rate of prediabetes among the African American and European American subjects with parental type 2 diabetes in the POP-ABC study appears to be at least of the same magnitude as the rate among Pima Indians, the group with the world's highest prevalence of type 2 diabetes.[23,25–27] These data illustrate the importance of a family (particularly parental) history of diabetes as a susceptibility factor for dysglycemia.[28,29]

Behavioral predictors

The effects of sedentary behavior and dietary factors in promoting the risks of obesity and type 2 diabetes have been well described,[30–33] but few studies have specifically focused on prediabetes. Dietary habits were recorded using the Food Habits Questionnaire, and leisure-time physical activity was captured using the Modifiable Activity Questionnaire in 338 normoglycemic subjects (mean age 45.2 ± 10.2 years, BMI 30.3 ± 7.2 kg/m^2).[33] The Food Habits Questionnaire and Modifiable Activity Questionnaire scores were individually correlated with BMI and waist circumference, indicating congruency between self-reported behavioral data and objective measures of adiposity.[34] During 5.5 years of follow-up, 101 subjects (progressors) developed prediabetes and 227 participants maintained normoglycemia (nonprogressors) (11 subjects developed diabetes and were not included in further analyses). The Food Habits Questionnaire scores for self-reported dietary habits did not differ significantly between progressors and nonprogressors to prediabetes; however, the Modifiable Activity Questionnaire scores for leisure-time physical activity were lower by 30% in progressors than in nonprogressors.[34]

Thus, of the self-reported behavioral measures, physical activity, but not dietary recall, significantly predicted incident prediabetes in the POP-ABC study that followed participants for 5.5 years.[33] The Food Habits Questionnaire was used to explore dietary habits in five subdomains: *1*) modifying meats to make them lower in fat, *2*) avoiding fat as a seasoning, *3*) substituting high-fat foods with manufactured lower-fat foods, *4*) augmenting diet with fruits or vegetables, and *5*) replacing high-fat foods with low-fat foods other than fruits or vegetables.[16] It is plausible that, while recall of such dietary habits correlated congruently with body weight, the instrument itself was less sensitive for the detection of dysglycemic risk.

Dairy consumption

A different instrument, the Food Frequency Questionnaire, was administered to 1,884 initially normoglycemic participants in the Framingham Heart Study Offspring Cohort, and data were analyzed in relation to incident prediabetes during a mean follow-up of 10.5 years.[35] After adjusting for age, sex, and energy intake, increasing consumption of dairy products was associated with a 37% lower risk of incident prediabetes.[35] However, total dairy and milk-based product intakes were not significantly correlated with baseline BMI or weight change, and the associations of dairy intake with incident prediabetes varied by dairy product and type and by baseline glycemic status.[35] The data for yogurt consumption showed a 25% reduction in the risk of prediabetes (versus nonconsumers) at a median intake of 1.7 servings per week, without further benefit above that amount.[35] The Framingham Offspring Cohort data are in accord with reports from studies in Brazil and Europe regarding the beneficial effects of diary and fermented dairy products on the risk of developing prediabetes.[36,37]

Yogurt and other fermented dairy products are thought to improve gastrointestinal, metabolic, and general systemic health through favorable interactions with gut microbiome.[38] In addition to their enhanced shelf life, fermented foods (such as cultured dairy products, bread, and fermented sausage) are valuable sources of micronutrients, vitamins, minerals, and antioxidants.[38] Importantly, the microorganisms responsible for fermentation as well as probiotics in fermented foods are now recognized as mediators of the health benefits associated with fermented foods. There is good evidence from epidemiological studies that links consumption of yogurt and other fermented foods to reduced risks of metabolic syndrome,[39] obesity,[40] and cardiovascular disease.[41] These association studies are supported by controlled clinical trials that demonstrate improved cardiometabolic outcomes after dietary supplementation with yogurt and other fermented foods.[42–45]

The molecular mechanisms of the health-promoting effects of the gut flora associated with consumption of fermented food products are currently under investigation. Omics techniques and next-generation sequencing help track the relative abundances of gut flora (such as firmicutes and bacteroidetes) associated with known cardiometabolic traits following consumption of a variety of fermented foods. Such information, along with characterization of the microbes present in fermented products, should yield a fuller picture of the interaction between the microbiome and human health.[39,46] The subject of gut microbiome and prediabetes risk is discussed further in Chapter 5.

Sugar-sweetened beverages, artificial sweeteners, and caffeine

Data from the Framingham Heart Study Offspring Cohort have shed light on the effects of habitual consumption of sugar-sweetened beverages (as compared with diet soda) on the progression of insulin resistance and development of prediabetes.[47] In that study, cumulative consumption of sugar-sweetened beverages or diet soda was analyzed in relation to incident prediabetes during 14 years of follow-up in 1,685 adults (mean age 51.9 ± 9.2 years; BMI 26.3 ± 4.4 kg/m^2) who had normoglycemia at baseline. There was no association between diet soda intake and risk of prediabetes, but intake of sugar-sweetened beverages was significantly associated with incident prediabetes.[47] Consumption of three or more servings per week of sugar-sweetened beverages was associated with a 46% higher risk of developing prediabetes compared with nonconsumers of sugar-sweetened beverages, after adjusting for BMI and multiple other confounders (adjusted hazard ratio 1.46, 95% CI 1.16–1.83).[47] In a related analysis of 2,076 participants from the same cohort who had serial measures of insulin resistance (homeostasis model assessment–insulin resistance [HOMA-IR]) for 7 years, higher consumption of sugar-sweetened beverages was significantly associated with a greater increase in HOMA-IR, after adjusting for BMI.[47] A previous report from the Framingham Offspring Cohort also showed an association between intake of sugar-sweetened beverages and increased risk of incident prediabetes (impaired fasting glucose) and metabolic syndrome during a mean follow-up period of 4 years.[48] Thus, insulin resistance appears to be a probable mechanism for the dysglycemia associated with sugar-sweetened beverages.

The epidemiological reports of the association between consumption of sugar-sweetened beverages and glucose dysregulation have been inconsistent[49–53]; however, a meta-analysis of 25 studies yielded an estimate that intake of one to two servings per day of sugar-sweetened beverages is associated with an 18–26% increased risk of developing type 2 diabetes.[54]

The literature on the possible association between intake of diet soda and glucoregulation is conflicting, with reports suggesting no effect on insulin sensitivity or increased risks of weight gain and insulin resistance.[47,55] The putative association between artificial sweeteners (contained in diet soda) and risk of type 2 diabetes has been investigated in epidemiological studies, with conflicting reports.[56,57] de Koning et al.[58] analyzed the self-reported consumption of sugar-sweetened beverages (sodas, fruit punches, lemonades, fruit drinks) or artificially sweetened beverages (diet sodas, diet drinks) in relation to the risk of type 2 diabetes among 40,389 men enrolled in the prospective Health Professionals Follow-Up Study cohort. Type 2 diabetes was diagnosed in 2,680 participants during 20 years of follow-up. When comparing men at the top quartile with the bottom quartile of sugar-sweetened beverage consumption, the age-adjusted hazard ratio for incident type 2 diabetes was 1.25 (95% CI 1.11–1.39, P for trend <0.01), but no significant risk was found after adjustments for family history, triglycerides, blood pressure, use of diuretics, BMI, weight change, and several other confounders.[56]

In line with emerging epidemiological studies[59,60] reporting favorable metabolic associations with caffeine consumption, de Koning et al.[58] observed that replacement of one serving of sugar-sweetened beverage with 1 cup of coffee was associated with a 17% reduction in the risk of developing type 2 diabetes. It is unclear whether the risk reduction resulted from the direct effects of caffeine or replacement of a sugar-sweetened beverage. However, there is a strong epidemiological association between regular coffee consumption (3–4 cups a day) and decreased risks of obesity, prediabetes, and type 2 diabetes.[59,60] Some proposed mechanisms for the beneficial properties of coffee included the effects of caffeine on insulin sensitivity and other putative health-promoting actions of chlorogenic acids.[59,61]

Clearly, in the management of patients with obesity and diabetes, replacement of sugar with artificial sweeteners is a prudent strategy for calorie reduction, and their use is in line with the scientific statement from the American Diabetes Association, the American Heart Association, and several other leading organizations.[62] A similar approach seems prudent for overweight or obese individuals with prediabetes.

References

1. Weyer C, Tataranni PA, Bogardus C, Pratley RE. Insulin resistance and insulin secretory dysfunction are independent predictors of worsening of glucose tolerance during each stage of type 2 diabetes development. *Diabetes Care* 2001;24:89–94
2. Weyer C, Bogardus C, Mott DM, Pratley R. The natural history of insulin secretory dysfunction and insulin resistance in the pathogenesis of type 2 diabetes mellitus. *J Clin Invest* 1999;104:787–794
3. Meigs JB, Muller DC, Nathan DM, et al.; Baltimore Longitudinal Study of Aging. The natural history of progression from normal glucose tolerance to type 2 diabetes in the Baltimore Longitudinal Study of Aging. *Diabetes* 2003;52:1475–1484
4. Li S, Xiao J, Ji L, et al.; China National Diabetes and Metabolic Disorders Study Investigators. BMI and waist circumference are associated with impaired glucose metabolism and type 2 diabetes in normal weight Chinese adults. *J Diabetes Complications* 2014;28:470–476
5. Orisaka M, Nakai K, Tominaga M, Suwabe A. Risk factors for development of pre-diabetic state from normal glucose regulation. *Tohoku J Exp Med* 2006;210:279–283
6. Dagogo-Jack S, Edeoga C, Nyenwe E, et al. Pathobiology of Prediabetes in a Biracial Cohort (POP-ABC): design and methods. *Ethn Dis* 2011;21:33–39
7. Dagogo-Jack S, Edeoga E, Ebenibo S, Chapp-Jumbo E. Pathobiology of Prediabetes in a Biracial Cohort (POP-ABC) study: baseline characteristics of enrolled subjects. *J Clin Endocrinol Metab* 2013;98:120–128
8. Dagogo-Jack S, Edeoga C, Ebenibo S, et al. Lack of racial disparity in incident prediabetes and glycemic progression among black and white offspring of parents with type 2 diabetes: the Pathobiology of Prediabetes in a Biracial Cohort (POP-ABC) study. *J Clin Endocrinol Metab* 2014;99: 1078–1087

9. Cowie CC, Rust KF, Byrd-Holt DD, et al. Prevalence of diabetes and impaired fasting glucose in adults in the US population: National Health and Nutrition Examination Survey 1999–2002. *Diabetes Care* 2006;29: 1263–1268
10. Cowie CC, Rust KF, Ford ES, et al. Full accounting of diabetes and pre-diabetes in the US population in 1988–1994 and 2005–2006. *Diabetes Care* 2009;32:287–294
11. Centers for Disease Control and Prevention. National Center for Health Statistics: National Health and Nutrition Examination Survey 2005–2006. Available from https://wwwn.cdc.gov/Nchs/Nhanes/2005-2006/DIQ_D.htm. Accessed 10 May 2021
12. Perreault L, Ma Y, Dagogo-Jack S, et al. Sex differences in diabetes risk and the effect of intensive lifestyle modification in the Diabetes Prevention Program. *Diabetes Care* 2008;31:1416–1421
13. Meigs JB, Cupples LA, Wilson PW. Parental transmission of type 2 diabetes: the Framingham Offspring Study. *Diabetes* 2000;49:2201–2207
14. Rung J, Cauchi S, Albrechtsen A, et al. Genetic variant near *IRS1* is associated with type 2 diabetes, insulin resistance and hyperinsulinaemia. *Nat Genet* 2009;41:1110–1115
15. Centers for Disease Control and Prevention. *National Diabetes Statistics Report, 2017*. Atlanta, GA, Centers for Disease Control and Prevention, U.S. Department of Health and Human Services, 2017. Available from https://www.cdc.gov/diabetes/data/statistics/statistics-report.html. Accessed 30 January 2020
16. Knowler WC, Barrett-Connor E, Fowler SE, et al. Reduction in the incidence of type 2 diabetes with lifestyle intervention or metformin. *N Engl J Med* 2002;346:393–403
17. Centers for Disease Control and Prevention. National diabetes fact sheet, 2011: diagnosed and undiagnosed diabetes in the United States, all ages, 2010. Available from http://www.cdc.gov/diabetes/pubs/estimates11.htm. Accessed 30 January 2020
18. Centers for Disease Control and Prevention. National Health Interview Survey (NHIS). Available from http://www.cdc.gov/nchs/nhis.htm. Accessed 30 January 2020
19. Benjamin SM, Valdez R, Geiss LS, et al. Estimated number of adults with prediabetes in the US in 2000: opportunities for prevention. *Diabetes Care* 2003;26:645–649
20. Williams DE, Cadwell BL, Cheng YJ, et al. Prevalence of impaired fasting glucose and its relationship with cardiovascular disease risk factors in US adolescents, 1999–2000. *Pediatrics* 2005;116:1122–1126

21. Lillioja S, Bogardus C. Obesity and insulin resistance: lessons learned from the Pima Indians. *Diabet Metab Rev* 1988;4:517–540
22. Ohlson LO, Larsson B, Svardsudd K, et al. The influence of body fat distribution on the incidence of diabetes mellitus: 13.5 years of follow-up of the participants in the study of men born in 1913. *Diabetes* 1985;34: 1055–1058
23. Knowler WC, Pettitt DJ, Saad MF, Bennett PH. Diabetes mellitus in the Pima Indians: incidence, risk factors and pathogenesis. *Diabetes Metab Rev* 1990;6:1–27
24. Abu Al Hommos N, Ebenibo S, Edeoga C, Dagogo-Jack S. Trajectories of body weight and fat mass in relation to incident prediabetes in a biracial cohort of free-living adults. *J Endocr Soc 2020*; bvaa164, https://doi.org/10.1210/jendso/bvaa164
25. Knowler WC, Pettitt DJ, Savage PJ, Bennett PH. Diabetes incidence in Pima Indians: contributions of obesity and parental diabetes. *Am J Epidemiol* 1981;113:144–156
26. Knowler WC, Pettitt DJ, Saad MF, Bennett PH. Diabetes mellitus in the Pima Indians: incidence, risk factors and pathogenesis. *Diabetes Metab Rev* 1990;6:1–27
27. Baier LJ, Hanson RL. Genetic studies of the etiology of type 2 diabetes in Pima Indians: hunting for pieces to a complicated puzzle. *Diabetes* 2004;53:1181–1186
28. Granner DK, O'Brien RM. Molecular physiology and genetics of NIDDM. *Diabetes Care* 1992;15:369–388
29. Willemsen G, Ward KJ, Bell CG, et al. The concordance and heritability of type 2 diabetes in 34,166 twin pairs from international twin registers: the Discordant Twin (DISCOTWIN) Consortium. *Twin Res Hum Genet* 2015;18:762–771
30. Gennuso KP, Gangnon RE, Thraen-Borowski KM, Colbert LH. Dose–response relationships between sedentary behavior and the metabolic syndrome and its components. *Diabetologia* 2015;58:485–492
31. Matthews CE, Chen KY, Freedson PS, et al. Amount of time spent in sedentary behaviors in the United States, 2003–2004. *Am J Epidemiol* 2008; 167:875–881
32. Thorp AA, Owen N, Neuhaus M, Dunstan DW. Sedentary behaviors and subsequent health outcomes in adults: a systematic review of longitudinal studies, 1996–2011. *Am J Prev Med* 2011;41:207–215
33. Mozaffarian D. Dietary and policy priorities for cardiovascular disease, diabetes, and obesity: a comprehensive review. *Circulation* 2016;133: 187–225

34. Boucher AB, Adesanya EAO, Owei I, et al. Dietary habits and leisure-time physical activity in relation to adiposity, dyslipidemia, and incident dysglycemia in the pathobiology of prediabetes in a biracial cohort study. *Metabolism* 2015;64:1060–1067
35. Hruby A, Ma J, Rogers G, et al. Associations of dairy intake with incident prediabetes or diabetes in middle-aged adults vary by both dairy type and glycemic status. *J Nutr* 2017;147:1764–1775
36. Drehmer M, Pereira MA, Schmidt MI, et al. Associations of dairy intake with glycemia and insulinemia, independent of obesity, in Brazilian adults: the Brazilian Longitudinal Study of Adult Health (ELSA-Brasil). *Am J Clin Nutr* 2015;101:775–782
37. Eussen SJ, van Dongen MC, Wijckmans N, et al. Consumption of dairy foods in relation to impaired glucose metabolism and type 2 diabetes mellitus: the Maastricht Study. *Br J Nutr* 2016;115:1453–1461
38. Kok CR, Hutkins R. Yogurt and other fermented foods as sources of health-promoting bacteria. *Nutr Rev* 2018;76(Suppl. 1):4–15
39. Babio N, Becerra-Tomas N, Martinez-Gonzalez MA, et al. Consumption of yogurt, low-fat milk, and other low-fat dairy products is associated with lower risk of metabolic syndrome incidence in an elderly Mediterranean population. *J Nutr* 2015;145:2308–2316
40. Sonestedt E, Wirfält E, Wallström P, et al. Dairy products and its association with incidence of cardiovascular disease: the Malmö Diet and Cancer Cohort. *Eur J Epidemiol* 2011;26:609–618
41. Mozaffarian D, Hao T, Rimm EB, et al. Changes in diet and lifestyle and long-term weight gain in women and men. *N Engl J Med* 2011;364: 2392–2404
42. Asemi Z, Samimi M, Tabassi Z, et al. Effect of daily consumption of probiotic yoghurt on insulin resistance in pregnant women: a randomized controlled trial. *Eur J Clin Nutr* 2013;67:71–74
43. Madjd A, Taylor MA, Mousavi N, et al. Comparison of the effect of daily consumption of probiotic compared with low-fat conventional yogurt on weight loss in healthy obese women following an energy-restricted diet: a randomized controlled trial. *Am J Clin Nutr* 2016;103:323–329
44. Nabavi S, Rafraf M, Somi M-H, et al. Probiotic yogurt improves body mass index and fasting insulin levels without affecting serum leptin and adiponectin levels in non-alcoholic fatty liver disease (NAFLD). *J Funct Foods* 2015;18:684–691
45. Ejtahed HS, Mohtadi-Nia J, Homayouni-Rad A, et al. Probiotic yogurt improves antioxidant status in type 2 diabetic patients. *Nutrition* 2012;28: 539–543

46. Tai N, Wong FS, Wen L. The role of gut microbiota in the development of type 1, obesity and type 2 diabetes mellitus. *Rev Endocr Metab Disord* 2015;16:55–65
47. Ma J, Jacques PF, Meigs JB, et al. Sugar-sweetened beverage but not diet soda consumption is positively associated with progression of insulin resistance and prediabetes. *J Nutr* 2016;146:2544–2550
48. Dhingra R, Sullivan L, Jacques PF, et al. Soft drink consumption and risk of developing cardiometabolic risk factors and the metabolic syndrome in middle-aged adults in the community. *Circulation* 2007;116:480–488
49. Austin GL, Krueger PM. Increasing the percentage of energy from dietary sugar, fats, and alcohol in adults is associated with increased energy intake but has minimal association with biomarkers of cardiovascular risk. *J Nutr* 2013;143:1651–1658
50. Aeberli I, Hochuli M, Gerber PA, et al. Moderate amounts of fructose consumption impair insulin sensitivity in healthy young men: a randomized controlled trial. *Diabetes Care* 2013;36:150–156
51. Faeh D, Minehira K, Schwarz JM, et al. Effect of fructose overfeeding and fish oil administration on hepatic de novo lipogenesis and insulin sensitivity in healthy men. *Diabetes* 2005;54:1907–1913
52. Le KA, Ith M, Kreis R, et al. Fructose overconsumption causes dyslipidemia and ectopic lipid deposition in healthy subjects with and without a family history of type 2 diabetes. *Am J Clin Nutr* 2009;89:1760–1765
53. Black RN, Spence M, McMahon RO, et al. Effect of eucaloric high- and low-sucrose diets with identical macronutrient profile on insulin resistance and vascular risk: a randomized controlled trial. *Diabetes* 2006;55: 3566–3572
54. Malik VS, Popkin BM, Bray GA, et al. Sugar-sweetened beverages and risk of metabolic syndrome and type 2 diabetes: a meta-analysis. *Diabetes Care* 2010;33:2477–2483
55. Gardener H, Moon YP, Rundek T, et al. Diet soda and sugar-sweetened soda consumption in relation to incident diabetes in the Northern Manhattan Study. *Curr Dev Nutr* 2018;2:nzy008
56. Nettleton JA, Lutsey PL, Wang Y, et al. Diet soda intake and risk of incident metabolic syndrome and type 2 diabetes in the Multi-Ethnic Study of Atherosclerosis (MESA). *Diabetes Care* 2009;32:688–694
57. Imamura F, O'Connor L, Ye Z, et al. Consumption of sugar sweetened beverages, artificially sweetened beverages, and fruit juice and incidence of type 2 diabetes: systematic review, meta-analysis, and estimation of population attributable fraction. *BMJ* 2015;351:h3576

58. de Koning L, Malik VS, Rimm EB, et al. Sugar-sweetened and artificially sweetened beverage consumption and risk of type 2 diabetes in men. *Am J Clin Nutr* 2011;93:1321–1327
59. Santos RM, Lima DR. Coffee consumption, obesity and type 2 diabetes: a mini-review. *Eur J Nutr* 2016;55:1345–1358
60. Mirmiran P, Carlström M, Bahadoran Z, Azizi F. Long-term effects of coffee and caffeine intake on the risk of pre-diabetes and type 2 diabetes: findings from a population with low coffee consumption. *Nutr Metab Cardiovasc Dis* 2018;28:1261–1266
61. Dewar L, Heuberger R. The effect of acute caffeine intake on insulin sensitivity and glycemic control in people with diabetes. *Diabetes Metab Syndr* 2017;11(Suppl. 2):S631–S635
62. Gardner C, Wylie-Rosett J, Gidding SS, et al.; American Heart Association Nutrition Committee of the Council on Nutrition, Physical Activity and Metabolism, Council on Arteriosclerosis, Thrombosis and Vascular Biology, Council on Cardiovascular Disease in the Young; American Diabetes Association. Nonnutritive sweeteners: current use and health perspectives: a scientific statement from the American Heart Association and the American Diabetes Association. *Diabetes Care* 2012;35:1798–1808

Chapter 4

Biochemical, Hemodynamic, and Inflammatory Predictors of Progression from Normal Glucose Regulation to Prediabetes

Glycemic and Glucoregulatory Predictors

During prospective follow-up of initially normoglycemic subjects, participants with higher baseline levels of fasting plasma glucose, 2-h plasma glucose (2hPG), and A1C progressed to incident prediabetes at a higher rate than individuals with lower values.[1,2] When baseline oral glucose tolerance test data were compared in initially normoglycemic subjects, some of whom later developed prediabetes during 5.5 years of follow-up, the levels of fasting plasma glucose and 2hPG emerged as significant predictors of incident prediabetes.[1,2] The mean fasting plasma glucose at baseline in progressors to prediabetes was 94 ± 7 mg/dL, compared with 91 ± 6 mg/dL in nonprogressors.[1,2] The mean 2hPG at baseline in progressors to prediabetes was 130 ± 27 mg/dL, compared with 121 ± 25 mg/dL in nonprogressors.[1,2] Thus, baseline fasting plasma glucose and 2hPG levels that fell within the upper half of the normal ranges identified individuals likely to progress to prediabetes during the ensuing 5 years. These findings are consistent with mechanistic studies that show a gradation of declines in insulin sensitivity and insulin secretion in relation to glycemia among individuals whose plasma glucose levels fall within the normal range.[3] Thus, the occurrence of upper-normal fasting plasma glucose and 2hPG could reflect a progressive shift in ambient insulin sensitivity and/or insulin secretion away from values that previously maintained lower, healthier levels of glycemia. Following that logic, the glucoregulatory defects precede the upward shifts in fasting plasma glucose and 2hPG. Alternatively, modest elevations in fasting plasma glucose or 2hPG can exert glucotoxic effects on insulin sensitivity and insulin secretion, thereby creating a vicious cycle.[4,5]

Consonant with glycemic measures, markers of glucoregulatory physiology, such as insulin sensitivity and insulin secretion, also significantly predicted progression to prediabetes in longitudinal studies.[1,2,6,7]

Insulin sensitivity

Weyer et al.[6] used the hyperinsulinemic-euglycemic clamp to document insulin sensitivity at baseline, at transition to prediabetes (impaired glucose tolerance), and at diagnosis of type 2 diabetes in Pima Indians and compared the data to serial changes obtained at equivalent time points in a control group who maintained normal glucose tolerance status throughout (nonprogressors).[6] Both low-dose (40 mU/m^2 body surface area per minute) and high-dose (400 mU/m^2 body surface area per minute) insulin-stimulated glucose disposal rates were lower at baseline in subjects whose conditions deteriorated from normal glucose tolerance to prediabetes (impaired glucose tolerance) compared with nonprogressors.[6] The low-dose insulin-stimulated glucose disposal decreased over time, but by a comparable degree, in both progressors and nonprogressors. However, the high-dose insulin-stimulated glucose disposal declined significantly by 12% during transition from normal glucose tolerance to prediabetes (and by 19% during further progression from impaired glucose tolerance to type 2 diabetes) but remained unchanged in nonprogressors.[6] The declines in insulin-stimulated glucose disposal were mostly attributable to decreases in nonoxidative glucose disposal (glycogen storage), whereas oxidative glucose disposal was largely unchanged during progression from normal glucose tolerance to higher glycemic states.[6] These findings are in accord with other longitudinal studies that found associations between lower baseline insulin sensitivity and increased risk of dysglycemia.[2,7–9]

Insulin-sensitive and insulin-resistant obese and lean phenotypes

Insulin sensitivity and overweight/obesity are closely related; however, dissociated phenotypes (insulin-sensitive obese or insulin-resistant lean) are being increasingly reported.[10–14] Owei et al.[15] measured insulin sensitivity with the hyperinsulinemic-euglycemic clamp in initially normoglycemic adults, to probe the existence of the subphenotypes of insulin-sensitive and insulin-resistant obesity and leanness, and their impact on the risk of progression from normal glucose regulation to prediabetes.[14] In that study, 320 healthy subjects (mean age 44.2 ± 10.6 years) underwent anthropometric measurements and assessments of insulin sensitivity at baseline, using the gold-standard hyperinsulinemic-euglycemic clamp method. Participants were stratified into *1)* insulin-resistant obese (BMI ≥30 kg/m^2), *2)* insulin-sensitive obesity (BMI ≥30 kg/m^2), *3)* insulin-resistant nonobese (BMI <28 kg/m^2), and *4)* insulin-sensitive nonobese (BMI <28 kg/m^2). During ~5 years of follow-up, insulin-resistant obese subjects developed incident prediabetes at a rate that was 56%

higher than that of insulin-sensitive obese subjects.[14] Strikingly, the risk of incident prediabetes was 80% higher among insulin-resistant nonobese subjects compared with insulin-sensitive nonobese subjects. Compared with insulin-sensitive obese subjects, insulin-resistant obese individuals harbored more cardiometabolic risk factors, as indicated by their higher levels of abdominal fat mass, serum triglycerides, and high-sensitivity C-reactive protein and lower levels of adiponectin.[15] Similarly, insulin-resistant nonobese individuals harbored more cardiometabolic risk factors than insulin-sensitive nonobese subjects, as indicated by their greater abdominal fat content, higher triglycerides and high-sensitivity C-reactive protein levels, and lower adiponectin levels[14] (Table 4.1).

The terms "metabolically healthy obesity," "metabolically benign obesity," or "insulin-sensitive obesity" are used interchangeably to refer to a phenotype of obesity that is associated with few (less than two) components of the metabolic syndrome.[10–14] Conversely, some normal-weight individuals express cardiometabolic risk by harboring two or more components of the metabolic syndrome and are referred to as "metabolically obese, normal weight."[16–18] Several reports have associated the metabolically healthy obese phenotype with a better cardiometabolic profile and decreased risk of type 2 diabetes compared to the metabolically healthy obese phenotype.[10–13,19–21] For example, in the Framingham Offspring Cohort study, insulin sensitivity (estimated using homeostasis model assessment–insulin resistance [HOMA-IR]) significantly distinguished individuals at risk of incident type 2 diabetes.[20] In a pooled analysis of eight prospective studies, the adjusted relative risk for incident type 2 diabetes was 2.2-fold higher in metabolically unhealthy obese subjects compared with metabolically healthy obese subjects.[21] Longer-term follow-up reports suggest that most metabolically healthy obese subjects may transition into an unhealthy phenotype, indicated by higher risks for type 2 diabetes, hypertension, and cardiovascular disease.[14]

Several mechanisms have been proposed to explain insulin-sensitive and insulin-resistant obese and lean phenotypes, but none provide full explanation. Suggested mechanisms include putative roles of visceral fat mass and hepatic enzymatic activity,[22] natural killer cells,[23] endocannabinoids,[24] expression of lipogenic transcription factors,[25] and mediation by higher adiponectin expression,[15,26,27] among others. In fact, the overexpression of adiponectin recapitulates the metabolically healthy obese phenotype in animal models.[28] The association between insulin-sensitive and insulin-resistant obese and nonobese phenotypes and the risk of type 2 diabetes has now been extended to prediabetes.[15] Thus, the emerging data support the incorporation of measures of insulin action in risk stratification and, possibly, for the targeting and timing of preventive interventions. The complexity of the hyperinsulinemic-euglycemic clamp method does make it unfeasible as a clinical tool in practice. However, there are less complex surrogate measures of insulin sensitivity, such as HOMA-IR, Matsuda Index, and QUICKI, all

Table 4.1—Cardiometabolic Profile of Insulin-Sensitive and Insulin-Resistant Obese and Nonobese Adults

Characteristic	IRO	ISO	*P*	IRN	ISN	*P*
Waist circumference (cm)	107 ± 11.9	102 ± 11.7	0.007	92.5 ± 8.10	81.7 ± 9.84	<0.0001
Total fat mass (kg)	42.2 ± 12.9	37.6 ± 10.6	0.015	24.5 ± 3.92	20.3 ± 6.10	0.009
Trunk fat mass (kg)	21.6 ± 6.49	18.8 ± 5.40	0.0032	13.1 ± 2.21	9.19 ± 3.12	<0.0001
SBP (mmHg)	127 ± 16.3	124 ± 15.5	0.16	123 ± 18.3	115 ± 12.6	0.03
DBP (mmHg)	75 ± 8.86	73 ± 8.60	0.19	78 ± 9.67	71 ± 8.43	0.009
HDL cholesterol (mg/dL)	48.8 ± 12.0	49.9 ± 10.9	0.54	44.8 ± 9.89	57 ± 14.9	0.0013
Triglycerides (mg/dL)	115 ± 57.7	89.7 ± 47.4	0.0019	134 ± 75.4	83.0 ± 48.8	0.0003
hs-CRP (mg/L)	6.34 ± 6.71	4.70 ± 7.15	0.013	3.06 ± 3.37	1.83 ± 2.65	0.08
Adiponectin (µg/mL)	7.38 ± 3.96	9.34 ± 4.46	0.003	6.56 ± 3.54	10.8 ± 6.02	0.006
HOMA-B (%)	158 ± 62.1	77.3 ± 41.3	<0.0001	132 ± 57.1	62.4 ± 62.7	<0.0001
AIR (µU/mL)	119 ± 91.9	84.3 ± 69.7	0.0061	135 ± 77.6	62.2 ± 52.7	<0.0001

IRO, insulin-resistant obese; ISO, insulin-sensitive obese; IRN, insulin-resistant nonobese; ISN, insulin-sensitive nonobese; AIR, acute insulin response to intravenous glucose; DBP, diastolic blood pressure; HOMA-B, homeostasis model of β-cell function (%); hs-CRP, high-sensitivity C-reactive protein; REE, resting energy expenditure. To convert the values for insulin to picomoles per liter, multiply by 7.175. To convert the values for HDL cholesterol to millimoles per liter, multiply by 0.02586. To convert the values for triglycerides to millimoles per liter, multiply by 0.01129.

derivatives of plasma glucose and insulin measurements during fasting or oral glucose tolerance tests.[3,29,30] Pragmatically, the waist circumference and the 2hPG during oral glucose tolerance test appear to integrate the dysglycemic risks conferred by ambient insulin resistance. In the Pathobiology of Prediabetes in a Biracial Cohort (POP-ABC) study, the hazard ratio (95% CI) for incident prediabetes for individuals at the 90th versus 10th percentile of the distribution for trunk fat was 2.9 (95% CI 1.74–4.82, $P < 0.0001$).[2] The hazard ratio for incident prediabetes for individuals at the 90th versus 10th percentile of the distribution for 2hPG was 2.54 (95% CI 1.46–4.40, $P = 0.0009$).[2] The combined hazard of having both trunk fat mass and 2hPG at the 90th versus 10th percentile was 7.35.[2] The waist circumference can be substituted for the trunk fat mass.[31]

Insulin secretion

Impaired insulin secretion is an early feature in individuals who develop type 2 diabetes and can be demonstrated before or during the prediabetes stage.[6,7,15,32–42] Serial measurements of fasting plasma insulin levels and insulin excursions at 30 and 120 min during an oral glucose tolerance test showed greater fasting insulinemia in the progressors to prediabetes than in nonprogressors.[6,7] The mean 30-min insulin levels during an oral glucose tolerance test (a measure of acute secretory β-cell function) did not change significantly from baseline during transition from normal glucose tolerance to prediabetes, but decreased by 24% during the transition from prediabetes to diabetes.[6,7] There were no significant temporal changes in the 120-min oral glucose tolerance test plasma insulin levels during transition from normal glucose tolerance to prediabetes or type 2 diabetes.[6,7]

Although fasting and oral glucose tolerance test plasma insulin levels yield information regarding glucoregulatory function, pancreatic β-cell insulin secretory function is more rigorously assessed using the frequently sampled intravenous glucose tolerance test (FSIVGTT). The FSIVGTT provides data for acute insulin secretory response to glucose (AIRg). Such rigorous assessments revealed that a lower baseline AIRg predicted progression to prediabetes,[6,7,15] and the AIRg decreased by 27% during the transition from normal glucose tolerance to impaired glucose tolerance (and by a further 51% during progression from impaired glucose tolerance to type 2 diabetes).[6,7] The control group of nonprogressors tested contemporaneously showed no early change in AIRg and a 30% increase at the time of final assessment, corresponding to occurrence of type 2 diabetes in the progressors.[6,7] The disposition index is a measure of insulin secretion that accounts for ambient insulin sensitivity. In support of the evidence for progressive decline in β-cell function, the disposition index decreased by 31.5%, during the transition from normal glucose tolerance to impaired glucose tolerance (and by an additional 47.5% during the impaired glucose tolerance to type 2 diabetes transition) in studies conducted among Pima Indians.[6,7] In the POP-ABC study, future progressors to prediabetes had 45% lower disposition index at enrollment compared with nonprogressors.[15] The 27% decrease in the AIRg during the transition from normal glucose tolerance to impaired glucose tolerance is evidence that impaired β-cell function is an early defect during the pathogenesis of type 2 diabetes.[6,7] The effect of early β-cell defect in the pathogenesis of prediabetes and type 2 diabetes is independent of insulin resistance.[7,31–33]

An interesting insight into the critical importance of insulin secretion was gleaned from a group of 15 subjects in the longitudinal Pima Indian study, whose glycemic status shifted from normal glucose tolerance to impaired glucose tolerance but later reverted to normal glucose tolerance during follow-up. It was observed that the transient worsening from normal glucose tolerance to impaired glucose tolerance was not associated with changes in the AIRg in those subjects. Thus, their ability to maintain insulin secretion (AIRg) predicted reversion from prediabetes to normoglycemia.[6] Similarly, in the Diabetes Prevention Program, greater insulin secretion at baseline was a significant predictor of regression from impaired fasting glucose/impaired glucose tolerance to normal glucose regulation during 3 years of follow-up.[43] Numerous mechanisms (including genetic factors, inflammation, glucose toxicity, lipotoxicity, amyloid degeneration, increased apoptosis, latent autoimmunity, and effects of drugs and toxins) have been proposed to explain the insulin secretory defect during the pathogenesis of dysglycemia[4,5,38–46] (Fig. 4.1). Postmortem studies show an ~30% decrease in β-cell volume in pancreatic islet cells isolated from individuals with antemortem prediabetes compared to control subjects with antemortem normal glucose tolerance,[42] consistent with the tandem findings of increased apoptosis.[42]

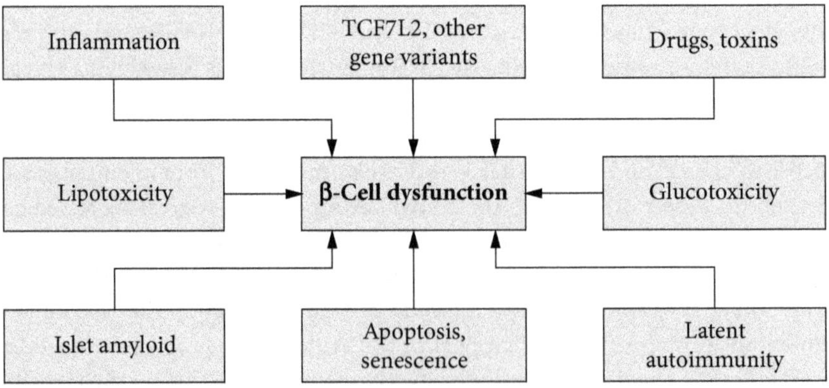

Figure 4.1—Mechanisms of β-cell dysfunction in the pathogenesis of prediabetes and diabetes.

References

1. Dagogo-Jack S, Edeoga C, Ebenibo S, Chapp-Jumbo E; Pathobiology of Prediabetes in a Biracial Cohort (POP-ABC) Research Group. Pathobiology of Prediabetes in a Biracial Cohort (POP-ABC) study: baseline characteristics of enrolled subjects. *J Clin Endocrinol Metab* 2013;98: 120–128
2. Dagogo-Jack S, Edeoga C, Ebenibo S, et al.; Pathobiology of Prediabetes in a Biracial Cohort (POP-ABC) Research Group. Lack of racial disparity in incident prediabetes and glycemic progression among black and white offspring of parents with type 2 diabetes: the Pathobiology of Prediabetes in a Biracial Cohort (POP-ABC) study. *J Clin Endocrinol Metab* 2014; 99:E1078–E1087
3. Dagogo-Jack S, Askari H, Tykodi G. Glucoregulatory physiology in subjects with low-normal, high-normal, or impaired fasting glucose. *J Clin Endocrinol Metab* 2009;94:2031–2036
4. Rossetti L1, Giaccari A, DeFronzo RA. Glucose toxicity. *Diabetes Care* 1990;13:610–630
5. Robertson RP, Olsen LK, Zhang H-J. Differentiating glucose toxicity from glucose desensitization: a new message from the insulin gene. *Diabetes* 1994;43:1085–1089
6. Weyer C, Bogardus C, Mott DM, Pratley R. The natural history of insulin secretory dysfunction and insulin resistance in the pathogenesis of type 2 diabetes mellitus. *J Clin Invest* 1999;104:787–794
7. Weyer C, Tataranni PA, Bogardus C, Pratley RE. Insulin resistance and insulin secretory dysfunction are independent predictors of worsening of glucose tolerance during each stage of type 2 diabetes development. *Diabetes Care* 2001;24:89–94
8. Meigs JB, Larson MG, Fox CS, et al. Association of oxidative stress, insulin resistance, and diabetes risk phenotypes: the Framingham Offspring study. *Diabetes Care* 2007;30:2529–2535
9. Tripathy D, Carlsson M, Almgren P, et al. Insulin secretion and insulin sensitivity in relation to glucose tolerance: lessons from the Botnia Study. *Diabetes* 2000;49:975–980
10. Ferrannini E, Natali A, Bell P, et al. Insulin resistance and hypersecretion in obesity: European Group for the Study of Insulin Resistance (EGIR). *J Clin Invest* 1997;100:1166–1173
11. Stefan N, Kantartzis K, Machann J, et al. Identification and characterization of metabolically benign obesity in humans. *Arch Intern Med* 2008; 168:1609–1616

12. Pajunen P, Kotronen A, Korpi-Hyövälti E, et al. Metabolically healthy and unhealthy obesity phenotypes in the general population: the FIN-D2D Survey. *BMC Public Health* 2001;11:754
13. Bluher M. The distinction of metabolically 'healthy' from 'unhealthy' obese individuals. *Curr Opin Lipidol* 2010;21:38–43
14. Echouffo-Tcheugui JB, Short MI, Xanthakis V, et al. Natural history of obesity subphenotypes: dynamic changes over two decades and prognosis in the Framingham Heart Study. *J Clin Endocrinol Metab* 2019;104: 738–752
15. Owei I, Umekwe N, Provo C, et al. Insulin-sensitive and insulin-resistant obese and non-obese phenotypes: role in prediction of incident prediabetes in a longitudinal biracial cohort. *BMJ Open Diabetes Res Care* 2017;5:e000415
16. Conus F, Rabasa-Lhoret R, Peronnet F. Characteristics of metabolically obese normal-weight (MONW) subjects. *Appl Physiol Nutr Metab* 2007;32:4–12
17. Wildman RP, Muntner P, Reynolds K, et al. The obese without cardiometabolic risk factor clustering and the normal weight with cardiometabolic risk factor clustering: prevalence and correlates of 2 phenotypes among the US population (NHANES 1999–2004). *Arch Intern Med* 2008;168:1617–1624
18. Ding C, Chan Z, Magkos F. Lean, but not healthy: the 'metabolically obese, normal-weight' phenotype. *Curr Opin Clin Nutr Metab Care* 2016;19:408–417
19. Kuk JL, Ardern CI. Are metabolically normal but obese individuals at lower risk for all-cause mortality? *Diabetes Care* 2009;32:2297–2299
20. Meigs JB, Wilson PW, Fox CS, et al. Body mass index, metabolic syndrome, and risk of type 2 diabetes or cardiovascular disease. *J Clin Endocrinol Metab* 2006;91:2906–2912
21. Bell JA, Kivimaki M, Hamer M. Metabolically healthy obesity and risk of incident type 2 diabetes: a meta-analysis of prospective cohort studies. *Obes Rev* 2014;15:504–515
22. Messier V, Karelis AD, Robillard ME, et al. Metabolically healthy but obese individuals: relationship with hepatic enzymes. *Metabolism* 2010;59:20–24
23. Lynch LA, O'Connell JM, Kwasnik AK, et al. Are natural killer cells protecting the metabolically healthy obese patient? *Obesity* 2009;17: 601–605
24. Osei-Hyiaman D, DePetrillo M, Pacher P, et al. Endocannabinoid activation at hepatic CB1 receptors stimulates fatty acid synthesis and contributes to diet-induced obesity. *J Clin Invest* 2005;115:1298–1305

25. Kantartzis K, Fritsche A, Machicao F, et al. Upstream transcription factor 1 gene polymorphisms are associated with high antilipolytic insulin sensitivity and show gene-gene interactions. *J Mol Med* 2007;85:55–61
26. Aguilar-Salinas CA, Garcia EG, Robles L, et al. High adiponectin concentrations are associated with the metabolically healthy obese phenotype. *J Clin Endocrinol Metab* 2008;93:4075–4079
27. Jiang Y, Owei I, Wan J, et al. Adiponectin levels predict prediabetes risk: the Pathobiology of Prediabetes in a Biracial Cohort (POP-ABC) study. *BMJ Open Diabetes Res Care* 2016;4:e000194
28. Liu M, Xiang R, Wilk SA, et al. Fat-specific DsbA-L overexpression promotes adiponectin multimerization and protects mice from diet-induced obesity and insulin resistance. *Diabetes* 2012;61:2776–2786
29. Matthews DR, Hosker JP, Rudenski AS, et al. Homeostasis model assessment: insulin resistance and beta-cell function from fasting plasma glucose and insulin concentrations in man. *Diabetologia* 1985;28: 412–419
30. Otten J, Ahrén B, Olsson T. Surrogate measures of insulin sensitivity vs the hyperinsulinaemic-euglycaemic clamp: a meta-analysis. *Diabetologia* 2014;57:1781–1788
31. Camhi SM, Bray GA, Bouchard C, et al. The relationship of waist circumference and body mass index to visceral, subcutaneous, and total body fat: sex and race differences. *Obesity (Silver Spring)* 2011;19:402–408
32. O'Rahilly SP, Nugent Z, Rudenski AS, et al. Beta-cell dysfunction, rather than insulin insensitivity, is the primary defect in familial type 2 diabetes. *Lancet* 1986;2:360–364
33. Pimenta W, Korytkowski M, Mitrakou A, et al. Pancreatic beta-cell dysfunction as the primary genetic lesion in NIDDM: evidence from studies in normal glucose-tolerant individuals with a first-degree NIDDM relative. *JAMA* 1995;273:1855–1861
34. Chen KW, Boyko EJ, Bergstrom RW, et al. Earlier appearance of impaired insulin secretion than of visceral adipocity in the pathogenesis of NIDDM. *Diabetes Care* 1995;18:747–753
35. Nagi DK, Knowler WC, Charles MA, et al. Early and late insulin response as predictors of NIDDM in Pima Indians with impaired glucose tolerance. *Diabetologia* 1995;38:187–192
36. Pimenta W, Mitrakou A, Jensen T, et al. Insulin secretion and insulin deficiency in people with impaired glucose tolerance. *Diabet Med* 1996; 13:S33–S36
37. Yoneda H, Ikegami H, Yamamoto Y, et al. Analysis of early-phase insulin responses in nonobese subjects with mild glucose intolerance. *Diabetes Care* 1992;15:1517–1521

38. Gerich JE. The genetic basis of type 2 diabetes mellitus: impaired insulin secretion versus impaired insulin sensitivity. *Endocr Rev* 1998;19: 491–503
39. Brunzell JD, Robertson RP, Lerner RL, et al. Relationships between fasting plasma glucose levels and insulin secretion during intravenous glucose tolerance tests. *J Clin Endocrinol Metab* 1976;42:222–229
40. Unger R. Lipotoxicity in the pathogenesis of obesity-dependent NIDDM: genetic and clinical implications. *Diabetes* 1995;44:863–870
41. Paolisso G, Tagliamonte MR, Rizzo MR, et al. Lowering fatty acids potentiates acute insulin response in first-degree relatives of people with type II diabetes. *Diabetologia* 1998;41:1127–1132
42. Butler AE, Janson J, Bonner-Weir S, et al. Beta-cell deficit and increased beta-cell apoptosis in humans with type 2 diabetes. *Diabetes* 2003; 52:102–107
43. Perreault L, Kahn SE, Christophi CA, et al.; Diabetes Prevention Program Research Group. Regression from pre-diabetes to normal glucose regulation in the diabetes prevention program. *Diabetes Care* 2009;32: 1583–1588
44. Moneva M, Dagogo-Jack S. Multiple drug targets in the management of type 2 diabetes mellitus. *Current Drug Targets* 2002;3:203–221
45. Hjort R, Alfredsson L, Andersson T, et al. Family history of type 1 and type 2 diabetes and risk of latent autoimmune diabetes in adults (LADA). *Diabetes Metab* 2017;43:536–542
46. Meier DT, Morcos M, Samarasekera T, et al. Islet amyloid formation is an important determinant for inducing islet inflammation in high-fat-fed human IAPP transgenic mice. *Diabetologia* 2014;57:1884–1888

Plasma Lipid Moieties and Incident Prediabetes

Elevated triglycerides and low HDL cholesterol levels are recognized risk factors for type 2 diabetes.[1] There is evidence that a similar risk relationship exists between dyslipidemia and prediabetes. Analyzing data from 335 normoglycemic adults enrolled in the Pathobiology of Prediabetes in a Biracial Cohort (POP-ABC) study and followed for ~5 years, baseline dyslipidemia was associated with increased risk of incident prediabetes.[2] In multivariate logistic regression models (after adjustment for age, sex, and BMI), higher baseline plasma levels of LDL cholesterol and triglycerides significantly increased the risk of incident prediabetes, whereas a higher HDL cholesterol level was associated with a significantly decreased risk of incident prediabetes. The relative risks (95% CI) of incident prediabetes were 1.97 (1.07–3.65) for LDL cholesterol, 1.63 (1.03–2.57) for triglycerides, and 0.46 (0.23–0.91) for HDL cholesterol. The combined relative risk of incident prediabetes for participants with lower baseline HDL cholesterol (10th vs. 90th percentile), higher LDL cholesterol (90th vs. 10th percentile), and higher triglycerides levels (90th vs. 10th percentile) was 4.12 (1.61–10.56).[2] Plasma lipid moieties correlated significantly with measures of adiposity, glycemia, insulin sensitivity, and secretion. Thus, baseline plasma lipid levels identified normoglycemic individuals at high risk for future glycemic progression to prediabetes. The exact mechanisms linking dyslipidemia and dysglycemia are not fully understood. Certain interventions that decrease cholesterol levels, such as statin therapy, have paradoxically been associated with increased risk for treatment-emergent type 2 diabetes.[3,4] On the other hand, other reports have suggested that the use of fibrates and statins may be associated with improved glucose tolerance[5] and decreased risks of diabetes and microvascular complications.[6–8] In fact, the bile acid sequestrant colesevelam, a drug initially approved as a lipid-lowering agent received expanded indication for diabetes treatment after demonstrating efficacy on glycemic control in a randomized controlled clinical trial.[9] Lifestyle modification in the Diabetes Prevention Program decreased triglyceride levels, raised HDL cholesterol levels, and decreased the incidence of type 2 diabetes.[10]

Baseline levels of HDL cholesterol and triglycerides had opposite correlations with insulin sensitivity and insulin secretion, which is a physiologically congruent finding.[2] Theoretically, improvement of insulin sensitivity probably via apolipoprotein A or HDL-associated mechanisms[11–13] can be expected to decrease insulin requirement, whereas triglycerides and their hydrolytic products (e.g., nonesterified fatty acids) induce insulin resistance.[14] A stimulatory effect of HDL on insulin secretion has also been shown in vivo[15] and in vitro,[16] providing yet another mechanism for the protective association between HDL cholesterol levels and incident prediabetes observed in the POP-ABC study.[2]

Unlike HDL cholesterol and triglycerides, LDL cholesterol levels are not substantially altered in patients with type 2 diabetes.[17] However, consistent with the observed association between higher LDL cholesterol and increased prediabetes risk among POP-ABC study participants,[2] studies in animal models have identified intra-islet accumulation of LDL cholesterol as a mechanism for β-cell dysfunction and glucose dysregulation.[18,19] The observation of a significant association between plasma lipids and the risk of prediabetes is supported by experimental and clinical data.[20–23] Elevations in circulating levels of nonesterified fatty acids and triglycerides precede the development of hyperglycemia in the Zucker diabetic fatty rat model.[14] Cross-sectional studies have reported associations between glycemia and plasma lipids, including the finding of higher triglycerides and lower HDL cholesterol levels in individuals with prediabetes.[22,23]

References

1. American Diabetes Association. 2. Classification and diagnosis of diabetes: *Standards of Medical Care in Diabetes—2020. Diabetes Care* 2019; 43:S14–S31
2. Owei I, Umekwe N, Wan J, Dagogo-Jack S. Plasma lipid levels predict dysglycemia in a biracial cohort of nondiabetic subjects: potential mechanisms. *Exp Biol Med (Maywood)* 2016;241:1961–1967
3. Ridker PM, Danielson E, Fonseca FAH, et al.; JUPITER Study Group. Rosuvastatin to prevent vascular events in men and women with elevated C-reactive protein. *N Engl J Med* 2008;359:2195–2207
4. Ridker PM, Pradhan A, MacFadyen JG, et al. Cardiovascular benefits and diabetes risks of statin therapy in primary prevention: an analysis from the JUPITER trial. *Lancet* 2012;380:565–571
5. Fulcher GR, Jones IR, Alberti KG. Improvement in glucose tolerance by reduction of lipid concentrations in non-insulin dependent diabetes mellitus. *Diabetes News* 1988;9:4–8
6. Flory JH, Ellenberg S, Szapary PO, et al. Antidiabetic action of bezafibrate in a large observational database. *Diabetes Care* 2009;32;547–551
7. Rajamani K, Colman PG, Li LP, et al.; FIELD Study Investigators. Effect of fenofibrate on amputation events in people with type 2 diabetes mellitus (FIELD study): a prespecified analysis of a randomised controlled trial. *Lancet* 2009;373:1780–1788

8. Davis TM, Yeap BB, Davis WA, Bruce DG. Lipid-lowering therapy and peripheral sensory neuropathy in type 2 diabetes: the Fremantle Diabetes Study. *Diabetologia* 2008;51:562–566
9. Bays HE, Goldberg RB, Truitt KE, Jones MR. Colesevelam hydrochloride therapy in patients with type 2 diabetes mellitus treated with metformin: glucose and lipid effects. *Arch Intern Med* 2008;168:1975–1983
10. Knowler WC, Barrett-Connor E, Fowler SE, et al. Reduction in the incidence of type 2 diabetes with lifestyle intervention or metformin. *N Engl J Med* 2002;346:393–403
11. Drew BG, Rye KA, Duffy SJ, et al. The emerging role of HDL in glucose metabolism. *Nat Rev Endocrinol* 2012;8:237–245
12. Han R, Lai R, Ding Q, et al. Apolipoprotein A-I stimulates AMP-activated protein kinase and improves glucose metabolism. *Diabetologia* 2007; 50:1960–1968
13. Drew BG, Duffy SJ, Formosa MF, et al. High-density lipoprotein modulates glucose metabolism in patients with type 2 diabetes mellitus. *Circulation* 2009;119:2103–2111
14. Randle PJ, Garland PB, Hales CN, Newsholme EA. The glucose fatty-acid cycle: its role in insulin sensitivity and the metabolic disturbances of diabetes mellitus. *Lancet* 1963;1:785–789
15. Briaud I, Kelpe CL, Johnson LM, et al. Differential effects of hyperlipidemia on insulin secretion in islets of Langerhans from hyperglycemic versus normoglycemic rats. *Diabetes* 2002;51:662–668
16. Fryirs MA, Barter PJ, Appavoo M, et al. Effects of high-density lipoproteins on pancreatic beta-cell insulin secretion. *Arterioscler Thromb Vasc Biol* 2010;30:1642–1648
17. Chahil TJ, Ginsberg HN. Diabetic dyslipidemia. *Endocrinol Metab Clin North Am* 2006;35:491–510, vii–viii
18. Kruit JK, Kremer PH, Dai L, et al. Cholesterol efflux via ATP-binding cassette transporter A1 (ABCA1) and cholesterol uptake via the LDL receptor influences cholesterol-induced impairment of beta cell function in mice. *Diabetologia* 2010;53:1110–1119
19. Tirosh A, Shai I, Bitzur R, et al. Changes in triglyceride levels over time and risk of type 2 diabetes in young men. *Diabetes Care* 2008;31:2032–2037
20. Liao C, Gao W, Cao W, et al. Associations of body composition measurements with serum lipid, glucose and insulin profile: a Chinese twin study. *PLoS One* 2015;10:e0140595
21. Chakarova N, Tankova T, Atanassova I, Dakovska L. Serum lipid and hsCRP levels in prediabetes: impaired fasting glucose (IFG) and impaired glucose tolerance (IGT). *Diabetes Res Clin Pract* 2009;86:56–60

22. Ganda OP, Soeldner JS, Gleason RE. Alterations in plasma lipids in the presence of mild glucose intolerance in the offspring of two type II diabetic parents. *Diabetes Care* 1985;8:254–260
23. Lee Y, Hirose H, Ohneda M, et al. Beta-cell lipotoxicity in the pathogenesis of non-insulin-dependent diabetes mellitus of obese rats: impairment in adipocyte-beta-cell relationships. *Proc Natl Acad Sci U S A* 1994;91: 10878–10882

Hemodynamics (Blood Pressure) and Incident Prediabetes

The Centers for Disease Control and Prevention estimates that 68.4% of U.S. adults 18 years of age or older with diabetes also have hypertension.[1] Etiologic factors for the occurrence of comorbid diabetes and hypertension include chronic kidney disease and rare endocrinopathies, such as Cushing syndrome. However, in most individuals with diabetes and hypertension who do not have nephropathy, the mechanisms linking the two conditions and their sequence of evolution remain unclear. Pathophysiologically, both hypertension and type 2 diabetes share common risk factors, such as obesity, physical inactivity, nutritional factors, and insulin resistance, among others.[2–4] Furthermore, both hypertension and type 2 diabetes display familial clustering and genetic predisposition. Although the gene variants reported to be associated with type 2 diabetes and hypertension are quite distinct, there are some overlapping loci that may provide a genetic basis for the shared risks of elevation of blood glucose and blood pressure.[5–8]

The development of hypertension or type 2 diabetes among initially healthy individuals is known to be preceded by the transitional stages of prehypertension and prediabetes, respectively.[9,10] Edeoga et al.[11] demonstrated that the well-known clinical association between hypertension and type 2 diabetes is preceded by a similar association between prediabetes and prehypertension.[11] After undergoing screening with an oral glucose tolerance test and blood pressure measurement, a total of 602 otherwise healthy adults were classified as having normal blood pressure, prehypertension, or hypertension, and normal glucose regulation, prediabetes (impaired fasting glucose/impaired glucose tolerance), or type 2 diabetes.[11] The subjects with normal glucose regulation were then enrolled in a 5-year prospective study, with the primary outcome of incident prediabetes. At baseline, participants with prediabetes were more likely to have either prehypertension (42.5 vs. 36.2%) or hypertension (21.6 vs. 15.2%) and were less likely to have normal blood pressure (35.9 vs. 48.6%) ($P = 0.009$).[11] The same pattern was seen among subjects with diabetes (Fig. 4.2*A*). Gupta et al.[12] analyzed blood pressure and blood glucose data from disease-free adult participants ($N = 4{,}561$) in the U.S. National Health and Nutrition Examination Survey (NHANES) 1999–2006 database. Similar to the findings by Edeoga al.,[11] the NHANES 1999–2006 data showed that individuals with prediabetes were more likely to have prehypertension and hypertension and less likely to have normal blood pressure than individuals with normoglycemia.[12]

During 5.5 years of follow-up of the normal glucose regulation group, Edeoga et al.[11] observed that the incidence of prediabetes was significantly higher among prehypertensive and hypertensive subjects compared with participants with normal blood pressure. Kaplan-Meier analysis showed a progressive decrease in prediabetes survival probability across the baseline blood pressure strata from normal

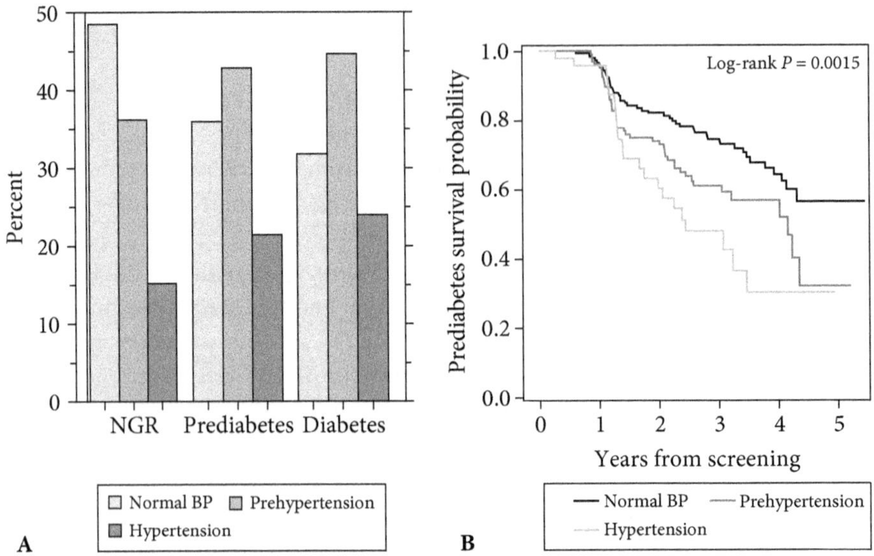

Figure 4.2—*A*: Prevalence of normal blood pressure (BP), prehypertension, and hypertension stratified by baseline glucose status. NGR, normal glucose regulation (as indicated by normal fasting plasma glucose and normal 2hPG during an oral glucose tolerance test (ANOVA $P = 0.009$). *B*: Kaplan-Meier plot of prediabetes survival probability among individuals with baseline normal BP, prehypertension, and hypertension during 5.5 years of follow-up.[11]

blood pressure to prehypertension to hypertension during 5.5 years of follow-up[11] (Fig. 4.2*B*). A linear correlation was observed between systolic blood pressure and both fasting plasma glucose and 2hPG values, and between diastolic blood pressure and fasting plasma glucose and 2hPG values.[11] Thus, baseline blood pressure status among initially normoglycemic individuals significantly predicted the occurrence of prediabetes 5 years later. That finding suggests that common or related proximal factors might be involved in the dysregulation of blood pressure and blood glucose and that the well-known clinical association between hypertension and diabetes had its origin long before the full-blown clinical expression of the blood pressure and blood glucose disorders.

It is plausible that shared environmental and genetic risk factors underlie the association of prediabetes and prehypertension and that the relationship represents a continuum toward the full-blown clinical end states of type 2 diabetes and hypertension. Indeed, certain gene variants have been associated with the phenotypes of hypertension and diabetes. Notable examples are ADRB3 (adrenergic β-3 receptor), CRH (corticotropin-releasing hormone), fibroblast growth factor receptor 1

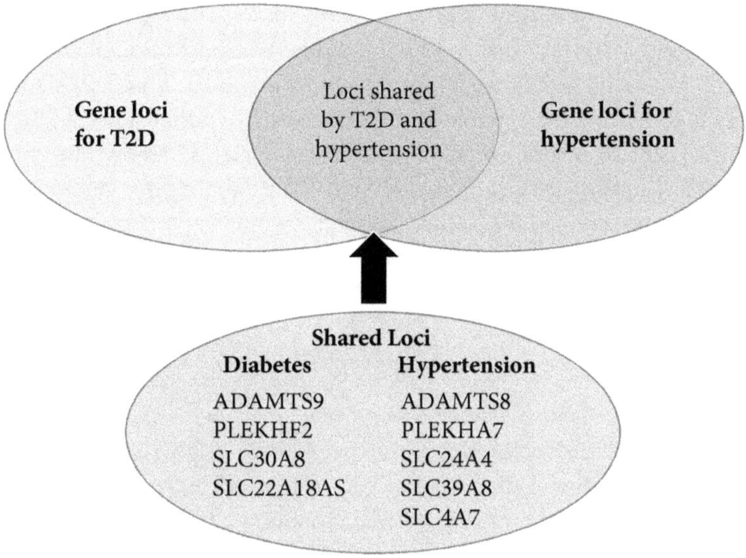

Figure 4.3—Overlapping loci for type 2 diabetes (T2D) and hypertension.[5-7]

(FGFR1), ADAMTS (a disintegrin and metalloproteinase with thrombospondin motifs), PLEKH (pleckstrin homology domain), and SLC (solute carrier).[5-8,13-15] ADRB3 is involved in catecholamine signaling and is a mediator of lipolysis and hemodynamic effects. CRH modulates metabolic and stress pathways; ADAMTS is involved in prohormone processing and vascular integrity; PLEKH is expressed in the pancreas; and SLC is a carrier for sodium and other solutes. Thus, although current functional understanding is incomplete, these gene variants do have congruent features that could have downstream effects on blood glucose and blood pressure (Fig. 4.3). Future exploration of such promising leads could help clarify the molecular basis of dual susceptibility to hypertension and diabetes.

At the environmental level, common behavioral factors (physical inactivity, overweight/obesity, and smoking) are well-recognized contributors to increased risks of hypertension and type 2 diabetes. Interventions that target these risk factors (including smoking cessation, increased physical activity, healthy eating pattern, and weight loss) could produce dual protection from future hypertension and type 2 diabetes among high-risk people with prediabetes and prehypertension. Data from the Diabetes Prevention Program indicate that lifestyle modification can simultaneously prevent progression from prediabetes to type 2 diabetes and decrease the incidence of hypertension, probably by preventing progression from prehypertension to hypertension.[16-18] Moreover, dietary intervention and increased physical activity improve blood pressure and blood glucose control in people who have developed hypertension and type 2 diabetes.[18,19] The reduction in the incidence of new-onset type 2 diabetes after bedtime administration of antihypertensive medications suggests that improvement in hemodynamic homeostasis can have a salutary effect on glucoregulation.[20] Currently, hypertension (but not prehypertension) is listed by the American Diabetes Association among the criteria for screening asymptomatic adults for diabetes or prediabetes.[21] Considering the emerging data, it is hoped that future guidelines would expand diabetes screening recommendations to include individuals with prehypertension.

References

1. Centers for Disease Control and Prevention. *National Diabetes Statistics Report, 2020.* Available from https://www.cdc.gov/diabetes/pdfs/data/statistics/national-diabetes-statistics-report.pdf Accessed 11 May 2021
2. Reaven GM. Relationship between insulin resistance and hypertension. *Diabetes Care* 1991;14(Suppl. 4):33–38
3. Natali A, Ferrannini E. Hypertension, insulin resistance, and the metabolic syndrome. *Endocrinol Metab Clin North Am* 2004;33:417–429
4. Long AN, Dagogo-Jack S. The comorbidities of diabetes and hypertension: mechanisms and approach to target organ protection. *J Clin Hypertens* 2011;13:244–251
5. Levy D, Ehret GB, Rice K, et al. Genome-wide association study of blood pressure and hypertension. *Nat Genet* 2009;41:677–687
6. Simino J, Rao DC, Freedman BI. Novel findings and future directions on the genetics of hypertension. *Curr Opin Nephrol Hypertens* 2012;21:500–507
7. Hivert MF, Jablonski KA, Perreault L, et al.; Diabetes Prevention Program Research Group. Updated genetic score based on 34 confirmed type 2 diabetes loci is associated with diabetes incidence and regression to normoglycemia in the Diabetes Prevention Program. *Diabetes* 2011;60:1340–1348
8. Dagogo-Jack S. Predicting diabetes: our relentless quest for genomic nuggets. *Diabetes Care* 2012;35:193–195
9. Vasan R, Larson M, Leip E, et al. Assessment of frequency of progression to hypertension in non-hypertensive participants in the Framingham Heart Study: a cohort study. *Lancet* 2001;358:1682
10. Meigs JB, Muller DC, Nathan DM, et al.; Baltimore Longitudinal Study of Aging. The natural history of progression from normal glucose tolerance to type 2 diabetes in the Baltimore Longitudinal Study of Aging. *Diabetes* 2003;52:1475–1484

11. Edeoga C, Owei I, Siwakoti K, et al. Relationship between blood pressure and blood glucose relationships among offspring of parents with type 2 diabetes: prediction of incident dysglycemia in a biracial cohort. *J Diabetes Complications* 2017;31:1580–1586
12. Gupta AK, Brashear MM, Johnson WD. Coexisting prehypertension and prediabetes in healthy adults: a pathway for accelerated cardiovascular events. *Hypertens Res* 2011;34:456–461
13. Magnusson M, Jujic A, Hedblad B, et al. Low plasma level of atrial natriuretic peptide predicts development of diabetes: the prospective Malmö Diet and Cancer study. *J Clin Endocrinol Metab* 2012;97:638–645
14. Avery CL, Freedman BI, Heiss G, et al.; Hypertension Genetic Epidemiology Network. Linkage analysis of diabetes status among hypertensive families: the Hypertension Genetic Epidemiology Network study. *Diabetes Care* 2004;53:3307–3312
15. Qu YY, Hui J, Wang LM, et al. Reduced expression of the extracellular calcium-sensing receptor (CaSR) is associated with activation of the renin-angiotensin system (RAS) to promote vascular remodeling in the pathogenesis of essential hypertension. *PLoS One* 2016;11:0157456
16. Knowler WC, Barrett-Connor E, Fowler SE, et al. Reduction in the incidence of type 2 diabetes with lifestyle intervention or metformin. *N Engl J Med* 2002;346:393–403
17. Diabetes Prevention Program Research Group. Impact of intensive lifestyle and metformin therapy on cardiovascular disease risk factors in the Diabetes Prevention Program. *Diabetes Care* 2005;28:888–894
18. Fuchs FD, de Mello RB, Fuchs SC. Preventing the progression of prehypertension to hypertension: role of antihypertensives. *Curr Hypertens Rep* 2015;17:505
19. Appel L, Moore T, Obarzanek E, et al. A clinical trial of the effects of dietary patterns on blood pressure: DASH Collaborative Research Group. *N Engl J Med* 1997;336:1117–1124
20. Dagogo-Jack S, Egbuonu N, Edeoga C. Principles and practice of nonpharmacological interventions to reduce cardiometabolic risk. *Med Princ Pract* 2010;19:167–175
21. Hermida RC, Ayala DE, Mojón A, Fernández JR. Bedtime ingestion of hypertension medications reduces the risk of new-onset type 2 diabetes: a randomised controlled trial. *Diabetologia* 2016;59:255–265

Inflammatory Signals and Prediabetes Risk

Proinflammatory signals

There are strong lines of evidence linking inflammatory markers with insulin resistance and increased risk of type 2 diabetes.[1–7] Using white blood cell count, a fundamental clinical measure of inflammation, higher levels have been shown to be predictive of incident type 2 diabetes.[1] In particular, higher granulocyte counts, but not lymphocyte or monocyte counts, have been specifically linked to the risk of type 2 diabetes.[1] Few studies have reported on white blood cell count and prediabetes risk, but there is a clear association between white blood cell count and markers of insulin resistance, even among normoglycemic individuals.[5] Besides white blood cell count, several molecular markers of inflammation have been associated with type 2 diabetes. Higher levels of proinflammatory cytokines (including C-reactive protein, tumor necrosis factor [TNF]-α, interleukin [IL]-6, IL-8, and fibrinogen) have been associated with insulin resistance, obesity, β-cell dysfunction, and increased risk of type 2 diabetes in experimental model and human studies.[1–7] In some reports, the odds ratio for incident type 2 diabetes in the upper quartile versus the lower quartile of the distribution of several proinflammatory cytokines is generally two- to three-fold or higher.[3,4] IL-1 has cytotoxic effects on pancreatic β-cells, and incubation with an IL-1 receptor antagonist, an endogenous inhibitor of IL-1 signaling, has protective effects on β-cells in vitro.[6,7] Incidentally, reduced serum levels of IL-1Ra were found in islet tissue from patients with type 2 diabetes, indicating an inherent loss of protection against β-cell damage.[7]

There is evidence that the association of cytokines with diabetes precedes the clinical development of diabetes and may represent a continuum of risk across glycemic thresholds. A number of cross-sectional studies have reported higher levels of proinflammatory cytokines in people with prediabetes compared with normoglycemic control subjects.[8–11] In the Diabetes Prevention Program, participants randomized to lifestyle intervention (who had a 58% reduction in risk of progression from prediabetes to type 2 diabetes) experienced an ~30% decrease in C-reactive protein levels from baseline to year 1 (compared to an increase of 5% in the placebo arm).[8] An even earlier-stage predictive relationship was observed in the prospective POP-ABC study, where higher baseline CRP levels were associated with increased risk of progression from normoglycemia to prediabetes during 5.5 years of follow-up.[11]

The mechanisms linking inflammation to increased diabetes risk include induction of insulin resistance and cytokine-mediated β-cell dysfunction.[1,2,12–15] Insulin-resistant states, such as polycystic ovarian syndrome, nonalcoholic steatohepatitis, and even hypertension, have all been associated with increased expression of proinflammatory cytokines.[16–18] The mechanism of the insulin resistance involves aberrant post-receptor insulin signaling: cytokines, such as TNF-α, are known to potently inhibit insulin-stimulated tyrosine phosphorylations on the β-chain of the insulin receptor and insulin receptor substrate-1 and divert post-receptor signaling from the normal tyrosine phosphorylation to phosphorylation of serine or threonine.[19,20] In animal models, inhibition of TNF-α results in improvement in insulin sensitivity through activation of insulin receptor tyrosine kinase in muscle and adipose tissue.[20]

Clinical interventions targeted at control of inflammation using hydroxychloroquine, salicylates, and monoclonal TNF-α antibodies have been reported to improve blood glucose control and prevent incident dysglycemia in patients with rheumatological disorders.[21–30] In a randomized controlled trial, treatment with salicylate (salsalate) decreased neutrophil counts and had no effect on high-sensitivity C-reactive protein levels, but significantly increased adiponectin levels and improved glycemic control in people with type 2 diabetes.[23] TNF-α inhibitors (such as adalimumab, certolizumab pegol, etanercept, golimumab, and infliximab), widely used for treating autoimmune and rheumatological disorders, have been reported to improve glycemic control in people with type 2 diabetes and sometimes induce hypoglycemia in people without diabetes.[25–29]

Similarly, treatment with a recombinant human IL-1 receptor antagonist, which decreased inflammatory markers, improved β-cell function and glycemic control in patients with type 2 diabetes.[30] The clinical finding that inhibition of inflammatory cytokines improves glycemic control strengthens the pathophysiological link between inflammation and glucoregulatory mechanisms. Additional support has emerged from the evaluation of new-onset diabetes among patients with rheumatoid arthritis receiving anti-inflammatory drugs. In a retrospective analysis, 1,127 adults with rheumatoid arthritis who had normal glucose levels were classified on the basis of whether they had ever used ($N = 333$) or never used ($N = 794$) hydroxychloroquine as part of their treatment regimen. A total of 48 patients developed incident type 2 diabetes during follow-up: three cases occurred in the group treated with hydroxychloroquine compared with 45 cases that occurred among the patients not being treated with hydroxychloroquine. The rate of new-onset type 2 diabetes was 6.2/1,000 person-years in the hydroxychloroquine group versus 22.0/1,000 person-years in the control group ($P = 0.03$).[21] These are intriguing results that bear confirmation in larger randomized, controlled prospective studies.

Adiponectin and prediabetes

In contrast to the diabetogenic association of proinflammatory cytokines, there is abundant evidence that higher adiponectin levels correlate with better cardiometabolic profile and decreased risk of type 2 diabetes.[31–34] The favorable cardiometabolic associations of adiponectin precede clinical diabetes and are evident at the prediabetes stage.[35–37] Banerjee et al.[37] compared fasting serum levels of adiponectin in age-, sex-, and BMI-matched groups of healthy subjects ($N = 52$), people with prediabetes ($N = 73$), or people with type 2 diabetes ($N = 77$). The authors observed that adiponectin levels were significantly lower in individuals with prediabetes (5.77 ± 1.6 μg/mL) or type 2 diabetes (4.96 ± 1.1 μg/mL) compared with healthy subjects (8.15 ± 2.6 μg/mL; $P < 0.001$) (37). Another case-control study also found significantly lower adiponectin levels in a group of 130 Jordanian subjects with prediabetes compared with 130 matched healthy control subjects; genotyping suggested a nominally significant association between a single nucleotide polymorphism (rs1501299) in the *ADIPOQ* gene and the risk of prediabetes.[38]

In a meta-analysis involving 3 cohort studies and 15 case-control studies (total sample 41,841 subjects), Lai et al.[39] reported that circulating adiponectin levels were 1.694 μg/mL lower (95% CI 1.237–2.151, $P < 0.001$) in prediabetes patients than healthy control subjects.

Among the participants in the Diabetes Prevention Program, all of whom had prediabetes at enrollment, baseline adiponectin level significantly and independently predicted the risk of progression to type 2 diabetes in the placebo, metformin, and lifestyle intervention groups.[35] To quantify the relationship, each ~3 μg/mL higher baseline level of adiponectin predicted a 39% reduction in the incidence of type 2 diabetes in the lifestyle group, a 24% reduction in the metformin group, and a 21% reduction in the placebo group.[35] Prospective follow-up data from the Diabetes Prevention Program showed that increases in serum adiponectin levels occurred in each of the treatment groups (more so in the lifestyle intervention group than the metformin or placebo groups). It was observed that every 1 μg/mL increase in adiponectin was associated with a 28% decrease in progression from prediabetes to type 2 diabetes in the lifestyle intervention group and an 11% decrease in the placebo group.[35] Among the Diabetes Prevention Program participants, weight loss was associated with increases in adiponectin in all treatment groups, particularly so in the lifestyle group. The protective effect of higher adiponectin levels persisted after adjusting for change in weight.[35]

The report by Mather et al.,[35] based on Diabetes Prevention Program participants, clearly documents the association between higher adiponectin levels and decreased risk of progression from prediabetes to type 2 diabetes. A report by Jiang et al.[40] extends observation to the more proximal stage of transition from normal glucose regulation to prediabetes, by analyzing data from normoglycemic individuals ($N = 333$) with parental history of type 2 diabetes (mean age 44.2 years) who were followed for the occurrence of incident prediabetes. Assessments at baseline included measurement of fasting plasma adiponectin levels: the mean level was 9.41 ± 5.30 μg/mL. Adiponectin levels in fasting plasma specimens obtained at baseline from the normoglycemic POP-ABC study subjects were inversely correlated with BMI, waist circumference, blood pressure, fasting plasma glucose, triglycerides, fasting insulin, HOMA-IR, and insulin secretion and were positively correlated with HDL cholesterol and insulin sensitivity.[40] During ~5 years of follow-up, 100 participants developed prediabetes.[40] Higher baseline adiponectin levels strongly predicted decreased risk of incident prediabetes (hazard ratio 0.48 [95% CI 0.27–0.86], $P = 0.013$).[40] Each 1-SD (~5 μg/mL) increase in plasma adiponectin was associated with a 52% decrease in prediabetes risk.[40] Thus, the well-known association of adiponectin with diabetes risk is evident at a much earlier stage in pathogenesis, i.e., during transition from normoglycemia to prediabetes.

Adiponectin is the most abundant secreted product of adipocytes, and its circulating levels are known to be positively associated with insulin sensitivity and strongly correlated with a favorable cardiometabolic risk profile.[31–34] Adiponectin has systemic anti-inflammatory, antioxidative, and insulin-sensitizing properties along with well-documented anti-apoptosis effects that protect pancreatic β-cells.[41] An interaction between adiponectin and fibroblast growth factor (FGF)-21 has been proposed as an important mechanism for the beneficial metabolic effects of adiponectin.[42,43] FGF-21 is a potent regulator of energy metabolism that improves insulin sensitivity and glucose tolerance in rodent models via upregulation of adiponectin expression.[43] FGF-21 promotes the clearance of toxic ceramides in obese animals, a process that is mediated by adiponectin-induced ceramidase activity.[44] Mice with targeted deletion of the adiponectin gene are refractory to the ceramide-clearing effects of FGF-21.[43] Tissue accumulation of esterified fatty acids promotes the biosynthesis of ceramides, a class of bioactive sphingolipids associated with the development of insulin resistance, diabetes, and cardiometabolic dysfunction.[45] Ceramides induce insulin resistance through activation of certain protein kinase C isoforms and disruption of key steps in the insulin signal transduction cascade.[45] Thus, through its interaction with FGF-21 and induction of ceramidase activity, adiponectin helps clear tissue accumulation of toxic ceramides.

The findings that a 5 μg/mL higher baseline adiponectin level predicted a 52% lower risk of progression from normoglycemia to prediabetes[40] and a 3 μg/mL higher baseline adiponectin level predicted a 20–40% lower risk of progression from prediabetes to type 2 diabetes[35] indicate that expression of high levels of adiponectin would preserve normal glucose regulation, whereas hypoadiponectinemia would be permissive of glucose dysregulation and increased risk of prediabetes and diabetes. These data indicate that adiponectin is a critical mediator of diverse cardiometabolic benefits. Thus, interventions that preserve or enhance adiponectin production should be valuable for cardiometabolic health. Such interventions include exercise (which can double adiponectin levels),[46] weight loss,[47] and smoking cessation.[48] As already noted, lifestyle (diet and

Table 4.2—Lifestyle Interventions and Medications That Alter Adiponectin Levels[45–59]

Increased adiponectin	
Lifestyle	
	• Exercise
	• Weight loss
	• Smoking cessation
Medications	
	• PPAR-γ agonists (thiazolidinediones)
	• PPAR-α (fibrates)
	• ACE inhibitors
	• Angiotensin II receptor blockers
	• Statins (variable effects)[52,53]
Decreased adiponectin	
	• Visceral obesity
	• Smoking
	• Glucocorticoids

exercise) intervention in the Diabetes Prevention Program increased circulating adiponectin levels, which independently predicted decreased risk of progression from prediabetes to type 2 diabetes.[35] Certain medications, including peroxisome proliferator–activated receptor (PPAR)-γ agonists (used for the treatment of diabetes),[49] PPAR-α agonists,[50] ACE inhibitors,[51] and angiotensin II receptor blockers[52] are also associated with increased adiponectin levels. Statins have been reported to have a variable effect on adiponectin levels.[53,54] Several of the interventions that increase adiponectin levels (e.g., exercise, PPAR-γ agonists, and ACE inhibitors) have been associated with decreased risk of diabetes and improved glucoregulatory outcomes in clinical trials[35,55,56] (Table 4.2). Weight gain, smoking, and treatment with insulin and glucocorticoids have all been associated with decreased adiponectin levels.[57–60] Of these factors, weight gain, glucocorticoids, and smoking are known risk factors for prediabetes/diabetes.

References

1. Shoelson SE, Lee J, Goldfine AB. Inflammation and insulin resistance. *J Clin Invest* 2006;116:1793–1801
2. Alexandraki K, Piperi C, Kalofoutis C, et al. Inflammatory process in type 2 diabetes: the role of cytokines. *Ann N Y Acad Sci* 2006;1084:89–117

3. Mirza S, Hossain M, Mathews C, et al. Type 2-diabetes is associated with elevated levels of TNF-alpha, IL-6 and adiponectin and low levels of leptin in a population of Mexican Americans: a cross-sectional study. *Cytokine* 2012;57:136–142
4. Liu C, Feng X, Li Q, Wang Y, et al. Adiponectin, TNF-α and inflammatory cytokines and risk of type 2 diabetes: a systematic review and meta-analysis. *Cytokine* 2016;86:100–109
5. Boucher AA, Edeoga C, Ebenibo S, et al. Leukocyte count and cardiometabolic risk among healthy participants with parental type 2 diabetes: the Pathobiology of Prediabetes in a Biracial Cohort study. *Ethn Dis* 2012;22:445–450
6. Bendtzen K, Mandrup-Poulsen T, Nerup J, et al. Cytotoxicity of human pI 7 interleukin-1 for pancreatic islets of Langerhans. *Science* 1986;232: 1545–1547
7. Maedler K, Sergeev P, Ehses JA, et al. Leptin modulates β cell expression of IL-1 receptor antagonist and release of IL-1β in human islets. *Proc Natl Acad Sci U S A* 2004;101:8138–8143
8. Haffner S, Temprosa M, Crandall J, et al.; Diabetes Prevention Program Research Group. Intensive lifestyle intervention or metformin on inflammation and coagulation in participants with impaired glucose tolerance. *Diabetes* 2005;54:1566–1572
9. Brannick B, Dagogo-Jack S. Prediabetes and cardiovascular disease: pathophysiology and interventions for prevention and risk reduction. *Endocrinol Metab Clin North Am* 2018;47:33–50
10. Kato K, Otsuka T, Saiki Y, et al. Elevated C-reactive protein levels independently predict the development of prediabetes markers in subjects with normal glucose regulation. *Exp Clin Endocrinol Diabetes.* 8 April 2019 [Epub ahead of print]
11. Dagogo-Jack S, Edeoga C, Ebenibo S, et al.; Pathobiology of Prediabetes in a Biracial Cohort (POP-ABC) Research Group. Lack of racial disparity in incident prediabetes and glycemic progression among black and white offspring of parents with type 2 diabetes: the Pathobiology of Prediabetes in a Biracial Cohort (POP-ABC) study. *J Clin Endocrinol Metab* 2014;99: E1078–E1087
12. Ye J. Mechanisms of insulin resistance in obesity. *Front Med* 2013;7: 14–24
13. Piao C, Wang X, Peng S, et al. IL-34 causes inflammation and beta cell apoptosis and dysfunction in gestational diabetes mellitus. *Endocr Connect* 2019;8:1503–1512
14. Catrysse L, van Loo G. Inflammation and the metabolic syndrome: the tissue-specific functions of NF-κB. *Trends Cell Biol* 2017;27:417–429

15. Saltiel AR, Olefsky JM. Inflammatory mechanisms linking obesity and metabolic disease. *J Clin Invest* 2017;127:1–4
16. Singh A, Amin H, Garg R, et al. Increased prevalence of obesity and metabolic syndrome in patients with alcoholic fatty liver disease. *Dig Dis Sci* 2020;65:3341–3349
17. Dunaif A. Insulin resistance and the polycystic ovary syndrome: mechanism and implications for pathogenesis. *Endocr Rev* 1997;18:774–800
18. Akash MSH, Rehman K, Liaqat A. Tumor necrosis factor-alpha: role in development of insulin resistance and pathogenesis of type 2 diabetes mellitus. *J Cell Biochem* 2018;119:105–110
19. Hotamisligil GS, Spiegelman BM. Tumor necrosis factor alpha: a key component of the obesity-diabetes link. *Diabetes* 1994;43:1271–1278
20. Solomon DH, Massarotti E, Garg R, et al. Association between disease-modifying antirheumatic drugs and diabetes risk in patients with rheumatoid arthritis and psoriasis. *JAMA* 2011;305:2525–2531
21. Bili A, Sartorius JA, Kirchner HL, et al. Hydroxychloroquine use and decreased risk of diabetes in rheumatoid arthritis patients. *J Clin Rheumatol* 2011;17:115–120
22. Goldfine AB, Fonseca V, Jablonski KA, et al.; Targeting Inflammation Using Salsalate in Type 2 Diabetes Study Team. Salicylate (salsalate) in patients with type 2 diabetes: a randomized trial. *Ann Intern Med* 2013;159:1–12
23. Kiortsis DN, Mavridis AK, Vasakos S, et al. Effects of infliximab treatment on insulin resistance in patients with rheumatoid arthritis and ankylosing spondylitis. *Ann Rheumatic Dis* 2005;64:765–766
24. van Eijk IC, Peters MJ, Nurmohamed MT, et al. Decrease of fructosamine levels during treatment with adalimumab in patients with both diabetes and rheumatoid arthritis. *Eur J Endocrinol* 2007;156:291–293
25. Wambier CG, Foss-Freitas MC, Paschoal RS, et al. Severe hypoglycemia after initiation of anti-tumor necrosis factor therapy with etanercept in a patient with generalized pustular psoriasis and type 2 diabetes mellitus. *J Am Acad Dermatol* 2009;60:883–885
26. Martínez-Abundis E, Reynoso-von Drateln C, Hernández-Salazar E, González-Ortiz M. Effect of etanercept on insulin secretion and insulin sensitivity in a randomized trial with psoriatic patients at risk for developing type 2 diabetes mellitus. *Arch Dermatol Res* 2007;299:461–465
27. Czajkowska JB, Shutty B, Zito S. Development of low blood glucose readings in nine non-diabetic patients treated with tumor necrosis factor-alpha inhibitors: a case series. *J Med Case Rep* 2012;6:5

28. Mastrandrea L, Yu J, Behrens T, et al. Etanercept treatment in children with new-onset type 1 diabetes: pilot randomized, placebo-controlled, double-blind study. *Diabetes Care* 2009;32:1244–1249
29. Larsen CM, Faulenbach M, Vaag A, et al. Interleukin-1-receptor antagonist in type 2 diabetes mellitus. *N Engl J Med* 2007;356:1517–1526
30. Kadowaki T, Yamauchi T, Kubota N, et al. Adiponectin and adiponectin receptors in insulin resistance, diabetes, and the metabolic syndrome. *J Clin Invest* 2006;116:1784 –1792
31. Goldstein BJ, Scalia R. Adipokines and vascular disease in diabetes. *Curr Diab Rep* 2007;7:25–33
32. Lindsay RS, Funahashi T, Hanson RL, et al. Adiponectin and development of type 2 diabetes in the Pima Indian population. *Lancet* 2002;360:57–58
33. Duncan BB, Schmidt MI, Pankow JS, et al. Adiponectin and the development of type 2 diabetes: the Atherosclerosis Risk in Communities Study. *Diabetes* 204;53:2473–2478
34. Mather KJ, Funahashi T, Matsuzawa Y, et al.; Diabetes Prevention Program. Adiponectin, change in adiponectin, and progression to diabetes in the Diabetes Prevention Program. *Diabetes* 2008;57:980–986
35. Liu C, Feng X, Li Q, et al. Adiponectin, TNF-α and inflammatory cytokines and risk of type 2 diabetes: a systematic review and meta-analysis. *Cytokine* 2016;86:100–109
36. Banerjee A, Khemka VK, Roy D, et al. Role of serum adiponectin and vitamin D in prediabetes and diabetes mellitus. *Can J Diabetes* 2017;41:259–265
37. Alfaqih MA, Al-Mughales F, Al-Shboul O, et al. Association of adiponectin and rs1501299 of the ADIPOQ gene with prediabetes in Jordan. *Biomolecules* 2018;8:117
38. Lai H, Lin N, Xing Z, et al. Association between the level of circulating adiponectin and prediabetes: a meta-analysis. *J Diabetes Investig* 2015;6:416–429
39. Jiang Y, Owei I, Wan J, et al. Adiponectin levels predict prediabetes risk: the Pathobiology of Prediabetes in a Biracial Cohort (POP-ABC) study. *BMJ Open Diabetes Res Care* 2016;4:e000194
40. Ye R, Scherer PE. Adiponectin, driver or passenger on the road to insulin sensitivity? *Mol Metab* 2013;2:133–141
41. Goetz R. Metabolism: adiponectin: a mediator of specific metabolic actions of FGF21. *Nat Rev Endocrinol* 2013;9:506–508
42. Holland WL, Adams AC, Brozinick JT, et al. An FGF21-adiponectin-ceramide axis controls energy expenditure and insulin action in mice. *Cell Metab* 2013;17:790–797

43. Reibe-Pal S, Febbraio MA. Adiponectin serenades ceramidase to improve metabolism. *Mol Metab* 2017;6:233–235
44. Mandal N, Grambergs R, Mondal K, et al. Role of ceramides in the pathogenesis of diabetes mellitus and its complications. *J Diabetes Complications* 2021;35:107734
45. Kriketos AD, Gan SK, Poynten AM, et al. Exercise increases adiponectin levels and insulin sensitivity in humans. *Diabetes Care* 2004;27:629–630
46. Yang WS, Lee WJ, Funahashi T, et al. Weight reduction increases plasma levels of an adipose-derived anti-inflammatory protein, adiponectin. *J Clin Endocrinol Metab* 2001;86:3815–3819
47. Kotani K, Hazama A, Hagimoto A, et al. Adiponectin and smoking status: a systematic review. *J Atheroscler Thromb* 2012;19:787–794
48. Yu JG, Javorschi S, Hevener AL, et al. The effect of thiazolidinediones on plasma adiponectin levels in normal, obese, and type 2 diabetic subjects. *Diabetes* 2002;51:2968–2974
49. Sahebkar A. Head-to-head comparison of fibrates versus statins for elevation of circulating adiponectin concentrations: a systematic review and meta-analysis. *Metabolism* 2013;62:1876–1885
50. Fontana V, de Faria AP, Oliveira-Paula GH. Effects of angiotensin-converting enzyme inhibition on leptin and adiponectin levels in essential hypertension. *Basic Clin Pharmacol Toxicol* 2014;114:472–475
51. Hass A, Oz H, Mashavi M, Shargorodsky M. Role of RAAS and adipokines in cardiovascular protection: effect of different doses of angiotensin II receptor blocker on adipokines level in hypertensive patients. *J Am Soc Hypertens* 2014;8:709–714
52. Li FY, Lam KS, Xu A. Therapeutic perspectives for adiponectin: an update. *Curr Med Chem* 2012;19:5513–5523
53. Chan KC, Chou HH, Huang CN, Chou MC. Atorvastatin administration after percutaneous coronary intervention in patients with coronary artery disease and normal lipid profiles: impact on plasma adiponectin level. *Clin Cardiol* 2008;31:253
54. Hanley AJ, Zinman B, Sheridan P, et al.; Diabetes Reduction Assessment With Ramipril and Rosiglitazone Medication (DREAM) Investigators. Effect of rosiglitazone and ramipril on β-cell function in people with impaired glucose tolerance or impaired fasting glucose: the DREAM trial. *Diabetes Care* 2010;33:608–613
55. Heart Outcomes Prevention Evaluation (HOPE) Study Investigators. Effects of ramipril on cardiovascular and microvascular outcomes in people with diabetes mellitus: results of the HOPE study and MICRO-HOPE substudy: Heart Outcomes Prevention Evaluation Study Investigators. *Lancet* 2000;355:253–259

56. Gariballa S, Alkaabi J, Yasin J, et al. Total adiponectin in overweight and obese subjects and its response to visceral fat loss. *BMC Endocr Disord* 2019;19:55
57. Kotani K, Hazama A, Hagimoto A, et al. Adiponectin and smoking status: a systematic review. *J Atheroscler Thromb* 2012;19:787–794
58. Fallo F, Scarda A, Sonino N, et al. Effect of glucocorticoids on adiponectin: a study in healthy subjects and in Cushing's syndrome. *Eur J Endocrinol* 2004;150:339–344
59. Shi JH, Du WH, Liu XY, et al. Glucocorticoids decrease serum adiponectin level and WAT adiponectin mRNA expression in rats. *Steroids* 2010;75:853–858

Chapter 5

Prediabetes: Insights from Genomics, Transcriptomics, microRNAs, Metabolomics, and Microbiomics

Genomics and Prediabetes

The heritability of diabetes has long been established through the studies of families and twins.[1–3] The field of monogenic diabetes illustrates the elegant utility of genetic techniques in identifying individuals with rare subtypes of diabetes and directing appropriate individualized therapy for patients with distinct types of maturity-onset diabetes of the young and neonatal diabetes.[4] Polygenic type 2 diabetes has also experienced explosive insights from the application of linkage analysis, candidate gene approach, and, more recently, genome-wide association studies to map its genetic landscape. Data from genome-wide association studies have enabled the identification of single-nucleotide polymorphisms (SNPs) at numerous loci.

Case-control studies comparing the frequencies of these SNPs enable calculation of the odds of their association with specific disease phenotypes. Such studies have discovered >40 variants or SNPs at numerous loci that are associated with increased risk of developing type 2 diabetes.[5–8] The diabetes-related SNPs identified to date individually confer modest effects. Most of the early work on risk information was obtained from European descendants, and there is always concern regarding possible allelic variation when applying the SNP panel to individuals of non-European ancestry.

Accordingly, performing replication studies in African American and other populations is prudent.[9,10] When assessing a panel of 17 diabetes susceptibility SNPs previously identified in European populations, Cooke et al.[9] reported significant diabetes associations for five SNPs at *ADAMTS9*, *WFS1*, *CDKAL1*, *JAZF1*, and *TCF7L2* among African American subjects. *ADAMTS9* is associated with tumorigenesis; *WFS1* encodes wolframin, a transmembrane protein expressed in pancreas, brain, and insulinoma β-cell lines; *CDKAL1* encodes a methylthiotransferase; and *JAZF1* encodes a zinc finger nuclear protein that functions as a transcriptional repressor. *TCF7L2*, the most replicated gene with SNPs that are strongly associated with type 2 diabetes, encodes a transcription factor in the *Wnt* signaling pathway.[11] *TCF7L2* is involved in β-cell survival and insulin biogenesis, among other putative functions.[11–13] Carriers of the *TCF7L2* risk allele manifest decreased glucose-stimulated insulin secretion and defective insulin processing.[11,12] Another highly replicated locus is the *CDKAL1*; association between diabetes risk and SNPs for *CDKAL1* has been replicated in European American, African American, British, and Asian populations.[5–10]

Interestingly, the majority of the SNPs described as conferring susceptibility to type 2 diabetes have functional implications that relate more to pancreatic growth, cell survival, insulin gene expression, and protein processing than insulin signaling. The SNPs associated with insulin secretory mechanisms and β-cell function include *ADRA2A*, *CAMK1D*, *CDKAL1*, *CDKN2A*, *CDKN2B*, *CENTD2*, *GCKR*, *GCK*, *GIPR*, *GLIS3*, *G6PC2*, *HNF1B*, *IGF2BP2*, *KCNJ11*, *KCNQ1*, *MTNR1B*, *NOTCH2*, *PROX1*, *SLC30A8*, *TCF7L2*, *THADA*, *WFS1*, and *SLC2A2*. By comparison, fewer loci have been associated with insulin signaling or impaired insulin action, as exemplified by *ADAMTS9*, *IGF1*, *IRS1*, *KLF14*, and *PPARG*. The *FTO* gene, due to its effect on obesity, can be added to the latter group[5–13,14] (Fig. 5.1).

Studies in ethnically diverse populations[9,10,13,15,16] have, so far, not revealed major ethnic-specific risk alleles that would explain the disparities in the prevalence of type 2 diabetes. For example, genome-wide association studies data from the multiethnic Diabetes Prevention Program cohort[15] indicate that the allelic frequencies of the *TCF7L2* risk variants (T = risk allele; c = other allele) are roughly similar in European American (TT 11%, Tc 45%, cc 44%) and African American (TT 10%, Tc 43%, cc 47%) participants with prediabetes. It is plausible that the discovery of more risk alleles from diverse populations might reveal novel informative markers through the recognition of rare alleles with major effects that are currently unknown. The latter notion is supported by the discovery of a previously unreported diabetes-associated gene variant in *ZRANB3* (zinc finger RANBP2-type containing 3).[17] To make that discovery, the investigators analyzed ~18 million autosomal SNPs in 5,231 study participants drawn from three sub-Saharan African populations (Nigeria, Ghana, and Kenya). The ZRANB3 risk alleles of genome-wide significance Chr2:136064024 (T allele) and rs1465146591 (A allele) had frequencies of 3.6% and 6.9%, respectively, in sub-Saharan African populations but are extremely rare in Europe, Asia, and the United States.[17] Functional studies in zebrafish and MIN6 β-cells (a mouse insulinoma cell line) demonstrated that the *ZRANB3* gene is a regulator of cell mass, apoptosis, and glucose-mediated insulin secretion in pancreatic β-cells.[17]

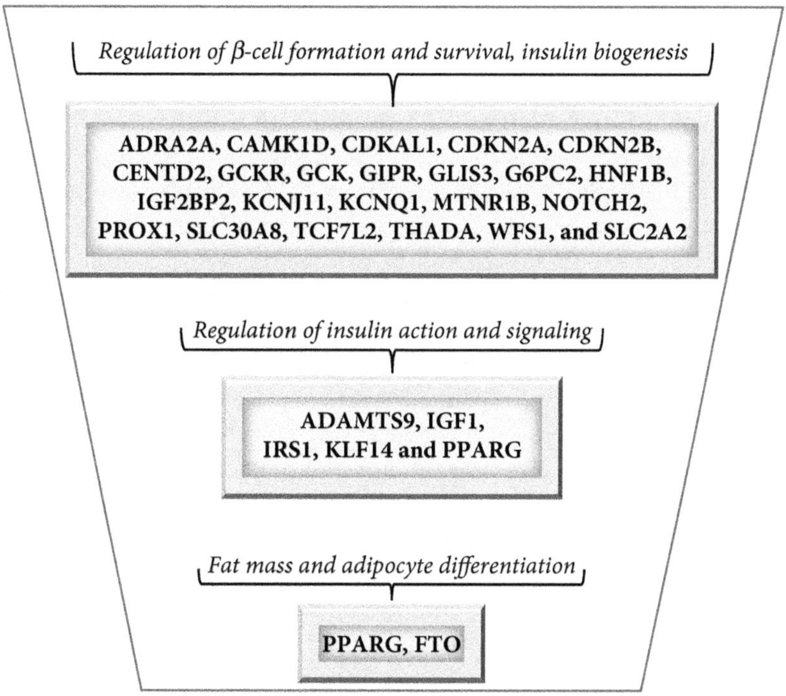

Figure 5.1—Gene variants associated with increased risk of type 2 diabetes clustered in functional groups related to β-cell and insulin biogenesis, insulin action, and fat mass and adipocyte differentiation.

Overall, the association of the individual gene variants (other than *TCF7L2)* with type 2 diabetes risk is rather modest in most studies, barely grazing nominal statistical significance in many instances. Chance associations become increasingly likely, especially with SNPs that are marginally significant in studies of limited sample size. A cumulative genetic risk score at several loci improves sensitivity. In the Diabetes Prevention Program cohort, 34 type 2 diabetes-associated variants were genotyped in 2,843 participants, all of whom had prediabetes at enrollment.[15] A genetic risk score was constructed by weighting each risk allele by its reported effect size on type 2 diabetes risk and summing up these values. The genetic risk score was then tested for its ability to predict progression from prediabetes to type 2 diabetes as well as regression to normal glucose regulation in adjusted models. The median weighted genetic risk score was 37.0 (range 23.7–51.5). The weighted genetic risk score predicted increased risk of progression from prediabetes to type 2 diabetes (1.02 per risk allele, $P = 0.03$) and decreased likelihood of reversion from prediabetes to normal glucose regulation, after adjusting for BMI, age, sex, ethnicity, and waist circumference.[15] Participants with a higher genetic risk score had worse β-cell function at baseline than participants who had a lower genetic risk score.[15]

The promise of genetic risk scoring for diabetes and other chronic disorders centers around three perspectives. First, the approach has the potential for robust prediction of diabetes risk. Second, it could enable the construction of targeted strategies for preventing, treating, or even curing the disorder (precision medicine). Finally, the increased knowledge could provide genomic clues to demographic differences in susceptibility to diabetes and its complications. Unfortunately, the available evidence does not support the promise of robustness in the prediction of diabetes.[18] For example, results from the Framingham Offspring Cohort study indicated parity between clinical risk assessment (using age, sex, family history, BMI, fasting plasma glucose, systolic blood pressure, HDL cholesterol level, and triglycerides) and genetic risk score derived from a cumulative genotype score at 18 loci regarding the ability to predict incident type 2 diabetes among normoglycemic subjects followed up for 28 years.[19] Similarly, genetic risk score at 34 loci did not add significantly to clinical risk factors in predicting incident type 2 diabetes among individuals with prediabetes during a mean 2.8 years of follow-up in the Diabetes Prevention Program.[15] Thus, the promise of robust prediction or facilitation of precision medicine, or of unraveling mechanisms of ethnic disparities, through genomic analysis, remains unfulfilled.

All Diabetes Prevention Program participants had prediabetes at enrollment, so it is important to determine whether it is the same type 2 diabetes-associated genes identified in the Diabetes Prevention Program, or different genes, that are involved in predicting progression to prediabetes among initially normoglycemic individuals. The natural history of untreated prediabetes is multidirectional: progression to type 2 diabetes, persistence of prediabetes, or reversion to normal glucose regulation. These spontaneous outcomes of prediabetes are regulated, at least in part, by genetic background.[15] It is plausible that a similar genetic regulation of the initial escape from normoglycemia to prediabetes exists. The rs7903146 variant in the *TCF7L2* gene is perhaps the best documented and strongest diabetes-related SNP. Individuals homozygous for the risk allele (TT) have a two-fold increase in the odds of having type 2 diabetes compared with those homozygous for the C allele.[20] Cropano et al.[16] performed an oral glucose tolerance test and genotyping of the rs7903146 variant in the *TCF7L2* gene in a multiethnic group of 955 obese children and adolescents, 307 of whom were restudied with an oral glucose tolerance test 3 years later. The baseline oral glucose tolerance test showed that 74% of participants had normal glucose tolerance and 26% had impaired glucose tolerance. The *TCF7L2* rs7903146 risk (T) allele was significantly associated with prevalent prediabetes (impaired glucose tolerance) among subjects from all ethnic groups studied, with odds ratios (OR) of ~1.60–2.0.[16] Carriers of the risk allele also had higher 2-h plasma glucose (2hPG) and decreased β-cell function.

Among 33 subjects studied with the hyperinsulinemic-euglycemic clamp along with isotope dilution techniques, the *TCF7L2* rs7903146 risk allele was associated with impaired suppression of endogenous glucose production, indicating either hepatic insulin resistance or incretin defect. Among the 307 subjects who underwent a follow-up oral glucose tolerance test, 202 subjects (66%) had normal glucose tolerance at baseline (*TCF7L2* genotype: 112 cc, 75 cT, and 15 TT), whereas 105 subjects (34%) had impaired glucose tolerance at baseline (*TCF7L2* genotype: 39 CC, 56 CT, and 10 TT).[16] During prospective follow-up, carriers of the T allele were more likely to progress from normal glucose tolerance to prediabetes (OR 2.648 [95% CI 1.326–5.291, $P = 0.005$]) and from impaired glucose tolerance to type 2 diabetes (OR 2.221 [95% CI 1.046–4.718, $P = 0.0379$]) compared with CC carriers.[16] The increased odds of incident prediabetes and diabetes during follow-up were independent of age, sex, BMI, changes in BMI, follow-up time, baseline 2hPG, and ethnicity.[16] Thus, this multiethnic study shows that harboring the rs7903146 variant in the *TCF7L2* gene conferred the same magnitude of risk of progression from normal glucose tolerance to incident prediabetes as it does for further glycemic deterioration from prediabetes to type 2 diabetes. That finding is consistent with the proposed mechanisms of the *TCF7L2* risk allele involving β-cell dysfunction.

The hepatocyte nuclear factor 4α (HNF-4α) P2 promoter polymorphism rs1884613 was also associated with increased odds of prevalent prediabetes, albeit in a Han Chinese population (OR 1.40 [95% CI 1.16–1.68, $P = 0.0001$]).[21] Because no association of HNF-4α rs1884613 with type 2 diabetes was observed in the same population, this SNP appears to be specific for prediabetes.[20] In a specific search for prediabetes-associated SNPs, Choi et al.[22] performed genome-wide association studies in healthy control subjects ($N = 3{,}153$) and individuals with prediabetes ($N = 2{,}529$) in Korea. The investigators identified two susceptibility loci associated with prediabetes: one at 17p15.3-p15.1 in *GCK* and another at 7p15.1 in *YKT6* (v-SNARE homolog). The rs2908289 in *GCK* and rs917793 in the *YKT6* gene were also significantly associated with microalbuminuria, after adjustment for age, sex, smoking history, systolic blood pressure, waist circumference, and serum triglyceride levels.[22] Previously, a common variant of the gene encoding a *GCK* regulatory protein was associated with protection against type 2 diabetes and chronic kidney disease.[23] *YKT6* is a soluble N-ethylmaleimide-sensitive factor attachment protein receptor (SNARE) that modulates synaptic-vesicle exocytosis. At present, there is no functional information regarding the association of the rs917793 variant in *YKT6* with glucose regulation or albumin excretion.

In conclusion, genome-wide studies have added valuable scientific data to current diabetes knowledge. However, the new information has not yielded a more robust prediction of polygenic type 2 diabetes than is achieved by common clinical and environmental risk factors. Furthermore, important functional information on most of the gene variants that appear to confer diabetes risk often is lacking, as is information on gene-gene interactions, gene-environment interactions, and correlative pathophysiological mechanisms. These limitations hamper the progress of genetic prediction and personalized intervention for the prevention and management of type 2 diabetes. The risk alleles in *TCF7L2* equally predict the risks of escape from normoglycemia and the subsequent progression from prediabetes to type 2 diabetes. Many of the other loci associated with type 2 diabetes could well emerge as signals in prediabetes if examined in carefully designed case-control studies. Most of the loci associated with increased type 2 diabetes risk appear to exert their effects via beta-cell dysfunction. Therefore, interventions that decrease insulin demand (by improving insulin sensitivity) can be expected to attenuate the diabetes risk associated with the gene variants. The latter realization adds to the complexity of gene-based prediction of diabetes risk.

References

1. Granner DK, O'Brien RM. Molecular physiology and genetics of NIDDM. *Diabetes Care* 1992;15:369–388
2. Willemsen G, Ward KJ, Bell CG, et al. The concordance and heritability of type 2 diabetes in 34,166 twin pairs from international twin registers: the Discordant Twin (DISCOTWIN) Consortium. *Twin Res Hum Genet* 2015;18:762–771
3. Moonesinghe R, Beckles GLA, Liu T, Khoury MJ. The contribution of family history to the burden of diagnosed diabetes, undiagnosed diabetes, and prediabetes in the United States: analysis of the National Health and Nutrition Examination Survey, 2009–2014. *Genet Med* 2018;20:1159–1166
4. Sanyoura M, Philipson LH, Naylor R. Monogenic diabetes in children and adolescents: recognition and treatment options. *Curr Diab Rep* 2018;18:58
5. Ehm MG, Karnoub MC, Sakul H, et al.; American Diabetes Association GENNID Study Group. Genetics of NIDDM: genomewide search for type 2 diabetes susceptibility genes in four American populations. *Am J Hum Genet* 2000;66:1871–1881
6. McCarthy MI, Zeggini E. Genome-wide association studies in type 2 diabetes. *Curr Diab Rep* 2009;9:164–171
7. Dupuis J, Langenberg C, Prokopenko I, et al.; DIAGRAM Consortium; GIANT Consortium; Global BPGen Consortium; Anders Hamsten on behalf of Procardis Consortium; MAGIC investigators. New genetic loci implicated in fasting glucose homeostasis and their impact on type 2 diabetes risk. *Nat Genet* 2010:42:105–116

8. Voight BF, Scott LJ, Steinthorsdottir V, et al.; MAGIC Investigators; GIANT Consortium. Twelve type 2 diabetes susceptibility loci identified through large-scale association analysis. *Nat Genet* 2010;42:579–589
9. Cooke JN, Ng MCY, Palmer ND, et al. Genetic risk assessment of type 2 diabetes-associated polymorphisms in African Americans. *Diabetes Care* 2012;35:287–292
10. Song C, Wang M, Fang H, et al. Effects of variants of 50 genes on diabetes risk among the Chinese population born in the early 1960s. *J Diabetes* 2019;11:857–868
11. Grant SF, Thorleifsson G, Reynisdottir I, et al. Variant of transcription factor 7-like 2 (*TCF7L2*) gene confers risk of type 2 diabetes. *Nat Genet* 2006;38:320–323
12. Saxena R, Gianniny L, Burtt NP, et al. Common single nucleotide polymorphisms in *TCF7L2* are reproducibly associated with type 2 diabetes and reduce the insulin response to glucose in nondiabetic individuals. *Diabetes* 2006;55:2890–2895
13. McCaffery JM1, Jablonski KA, Franks PW, et al.; Diabetes Prevention Program Research Group. *TCF7L2* polymorphism, weight loss and proinsulin:insulin ratio in the diabetes prevention program. *PLoS One* 2011;6:e21518
14. Gjesing AP, Pedersen O. 'Omics'-driven discoveries in prevention and treatment of type 2 diabetes. *Eur J Clin Invest* 2012;42:579–588
15. Hivert MF, Jablonski KA, Perreault L, et al.; Diabetes Prevention Program Research Group. Updated genetic score based on 34 confirmed type 2 diabetes loci is associated with diabetes incidence and regression to normoglycemia in the Diabetes Prevention Program. *Diabetes* 2011;60:1340–1348
16. Cropano C, Santoro N, Groop L, et al. The rs7903146 variant in the *TCF7L2* gene increases the risk of prediabetes/type 2 diabetes in obese adolescents by impairing β-cell function and hepatic insulin sensitivity. *Diabetes Care* 2017;40:1082–1089
17. Adeyemo AA, Zaghloul NA, Chen G, et al.; South Africa Zulu Type 2 Diabetes Case-Control Study. ZRANB3 is an African-specific type 2 diabetes locus associated with beta-cell mass and insulin response. *Nat Commun* 2019;10:3195
18. Dagogo-Jack S. Predicting diabetes: our relentless quest for genomic nuggets. *Diabetes Care* 2012;35:193–195
19. Meigs JB, Shrader P, Sullivan LM, et al. Genotype score in addition to common risk factors for prediction of type 2 diabetes. *N Engl J Med* 2008;359:2208–2219
20. Tong Y, Lin Y, Zhang Y, et al. Association between *TCF7L2* gene polymorphisms and susceptibility to type 2 diabetes mellitus: a large Human

Genome Epidemiology (HuGE) review and meta-analysis. *BMC Med Genet* 2009;10:15
21. Wang C, Chen S, Zhang T, et al. Prediabetes is associated with HNF-4α P2 promoter polymorphism rs1884613: a case-control study in Han Chinese population and an updated meta-analysis. *Dis Markers* 2014;2014: 231736
22. Choi JW, Moon S, Jang EJ, et al. Association of prediabetes-associated single nucleotide polymorphisms with microalbuminuria. *PLoS One* 2017;12:e0171367
23. Brouwers CGJ, Jacobs C, Bast A, et al. Modulation of glucokinase regulatory protein: a double-edged sword? *Trends Mol Med* 2015;21:583–594

MicroRNA Expression Profiles in Prediabetes

MicroRNAs (miRNAs) are short, noncoding RNA molecules that bind to the untranslated regions of target mRNAs and cause message destabilization (Table 5.1). Thus, miRNAs act as regulators of gene expression at the posttranscriptional level, principally by inhibiting translation.[1–4] More than 2,000 mature human miRNAs have been identified since the first miRNA was reported in the 1990s, and these small molecules (typically 22 nucleotides) have been implicated in the etiology of diverse neoplastic and benign disorders. Evidence is accumulating that the expression profiles of specific miRNAs may be associated with diabetes risk via mechanisms that include pancreatic islet β-cell survival.[5–7] Certain miRNAs (e.g., miR-375, miR-204, miR-184, and miR-503) have been reported to regulate pancreatic β-cell mass and function.[7–9] The overexpression of miR-142-3p in an insulinoma cell line (INS-1) stimulated cell proliferation and inhibited apoptosis.[10] Notably, miR-142-3p levels are upregulated in embryonic tissue and peripheral blood obtained from a mouse model of gestational diabetes,[10] and microRNAs are increasingly being linked to the adaptive expansion of β-cell mass in states of increased insulin demand, such as pregnancy.[11]

Multiple reports have observed altered patterns of miRNA expression in serum or plasma samples from patients with type 1 or type 2 diabetes compared to the pattern seen in healthy control subjects.[4,5,12,13] When comparing healthy subjects and patients with type 1 diabetes, differential expression of 11 circulating miRNAs (miR-21-5p, miR-24-3p, miR-100-5p, miR-146a-5p, miR-148a-3p, miR-150-5p, miR-181a-5p, miR-210-5p, miR-342-3p, miR-375, and miR-1275) was reported frequently.[12] Similar studies comparing patients with type 2 diabetes versus control subjects found discordant miRNA expression profiles involving scores of individual miRNAs.[13] In a meta-analysis, some 40 miRNAs were reported to be significantly discordant in patients with type 2 diabetes, among which miR-29a, miR-34a, miR-103, miR-107, miR-132, miR-142-3p, miR-144, and miR-375 appeared

Table 5.1—Properties of MicroRNAs (miRNAs)

- miRNAs are short, non-coding RNA molecules
- miRNAs typically have ~22 nucleotides
- The first miRNA was reported in 1990s
- >2000 mature human miRNAs currently identified
- miRNAs bind to the untranslated regions of target mRNAs
- miRNAs regulators gene expression at the post-transcriptional level
- miRNAs may play a role in the etiology of diverse neoplastic and benign disorders
- Specific miRNAs may be associated with increased diabetes risk

promising as emerging biomarkers of diabetes risk.[13] Notably, many workers have reported that miR-126a is consistenly downregulated in patients with type 2 diabetes and in people with impaired fasting glucose.[13,14] Furthermore, analyses of miRNA expression profiles in banked human islets have shown differential patterns (either overexpression or downregulation of certain miRNAs) in islet cells from people with type 1 or type 2 diabetes compared with healthy subjects.[12,15,16]

Emerging data indicate that individuals with prediabetes have a different profile of circulating miRNAs compared to individuals with normal glucose.[17,18] In one report, there was a progressive increase in the global quantity of miRNAs expressed in people with impaired glucose tolerance and type 2 diabetes compared to subjects with normal glucose tolerance.[17] A significant correlation was observed between global miRNA quantity versus plasma glucose and A1C levels, respectively.[17] The cross-sectional design of those studies does not permit inferences as to whether the increased levels of circulating miRNAs caused or resulted from progressive glucose dysregulation. Longitudinal studies are needed to tease out the chronology and direction of the association between miRNA expression patterns and glucose abnormalities.

Preliminary data from the prospective Pathobiology of Prediabetes in a Biracial Cohort (POP-ABC) study identified 25 miRNAs that were differentially expressed between individuals who progressed from normal glucose regulation to prediabetes and nonprogressors (Table 5.2).[19] The initially normoglycemic POP-ABC study participants (age 49.7 ± 5.42 years; BMI 28.6 ± 5.77 kg/m^2) were followed for 5 years for the primary outcome of progression from normoglycemia to prediabetes (impaired fasting glucose/impaired glucose tolerance). Baseline plasma specimens from a representative group of participants with incident prediabetes (progressors, $N = 10$) and a matched group of nonprogressors ($N = 10$) were analyzed for miroRNA expression. Using next-generation sequencing, >12 million reads per sample were performed, and false discovey error was minimized by using Benjamini-Hochberg corrected P values to assess differential miRNA expression. Based on entries in miRBase_20, a total of 226 known miRNAs were identified at expression levels of >1 tag per million, and 151 known microRNAs were identified at expression levels of >10 tags per million. From this pool, 25 miRNAs were differentially expressed in baseline plasma specimens from progressors to prediabetes versus nonprogressors ($P = 0.04$ to <0.0001). The five most upregulated miRNAs in progressors (vs. nonprogressors) were miR-216a-5p, miR-217, miR-211-5p, miR-149-5p, and miR-204-5p (log fold-change 3.61 to 6.49, $P < 0.0001$). The five most downregulated miRNAs in progressors (vs. nonprogressors) were miR-34c-5p, miR-550a-3p, miR-3200-3p, miR-144-5p, and miR-144-3p (log fold-change −2.26 to −3.79, $P = 0.0009$ to <0.0001). Comparing progressors versus nonprogressors to prediabetes, the most differentially expressed miRNA was miR-216a-5p, for which expression was 6.49 log-fold higher in progressors

Table 5.2—List of 25 Most Differentially Expressed MicroRNAs between Progressors to Prediabetes versus Nonprogressors during 5.5 Years of Follow-Up[19]

MicroRNA	Log Fold-Change*	*P*
hsa-miR-216a-5p	5.81	<0.0001
hsa-miR-217	4.30	<0.0001
hsa-miR-144-5p	–3.66	<0.0001
hsa-miR-19b-3p	–1.70	<0.0001
hsa-miR-144-3p	–2.71	<0.0001
hsa-miR-624-5p	–2.48	<0.0001
hsa-miR-149-5p	3.98	<0.0001
hsa-miR-1299	3.58	<0.0001
hsa-miR-190a-5p	–2.53	<0.0001
hsa-miR-16-1-3p	–3.04	<0.0001
hsa-miR-20a-5p	–1.59	<0.0001
hsa-miR-186-5p	–1.33	<0.0001
hsa-miR-19a-3p	–1.56	<0.0001
hsa-miR-378a-5p	–2.04	<0.0001
hsa-miR-15a-5p	–1.32	<0.0001
hsa-miR-454-3p	–2.21	<0.0001
hsa-miR-500a-5p	–2.59	0.0001
hsa-miR-181d-5p	1.15	0.0001
hsa-miR-20b-5p	–1.81	0.0001
hsa-miR-9-5p	3.08	0.0001
hsa-miR-218-5p	2.09	0.0001
hsa-miR-362-5p	–2.38	0.0001
hsa-miR-548d-5p	–1.41	0.0001
hsa-miR-550a-3p	–2.49	0.0001
hsa-miR-375	2.45	0.0001

*Expression in progressors/nonprogressors.

than nonprogressors.[19] A search of microRNA databases indicates that miR-216a-5p may be involved in the regulation of up to 577 genes (Table 5.3), including several genes that modulate pancreatic β-cell proliferation as well as glucose, lipid, endocrine, and metabolic pathways.[20] Pending confirmation in larger studies, the data from the POP-ABC study suggest that miR-216a-5p may be a novel biomarker of early dysglycemia.

Table 5.3—Some Target Genes of miR216a-5p Related to Metabolic Pathways (culled from a total of 577 genes)

Gene	Description	Evidence
PTEN	Phosphatase and tensin homolog (ENSG00000171862)	Experimental
SIRT1	Sirtuin 1 (ENSG00000096717)	Experimental
APOOL	Apolipoprotein O-like (ENSG00000155008)	Predicted
ATL3	Atlastin GTPase 3 (ENSG00000184743)	Predicted
ATP1B3	ATPase, Na+/K+ transporting, beta 3 polypeptide (ENSG00000069849)	Predicted
BMP10	Bone morphogenetic protein 10 (ENSG00000163217)	Predicted
CCNL1	Cyclin L1 (ENSG00000163660)	Predicted
CD200R1	CD200 receptor 1 (ENSG00000163606)	Predicted
CFL2	Cofilin 2 (muscle) (ENSG00000165410)	Predicted
CCNL1	Cyclin L1 (ENSG00000163660)	Predicted
COL9A1	Collagen, type IX, alpha 1 (ENSG00000112280)	Predicted
FMNL1	Formin-like 1 (ENSG00000184922)	Predicted
HINT1	Histidine triad nucleotide binding protein 1 (ENSG00000169567)	Predicted
HNF4G	Hepatocyte nuclear factor 4, gamma (ENSG00000164749)	Predicted
IKBIP	IKBKB interacting protein (ENSG00000166130)	Predicted
MTTP	Microsomal triglyceride transfer protein (ENSG00000138823)	Predicted
NGFRAP1	Nerve growth factor receptor (TNFRSF16) associated protein 1 (ENSG00000166681)	Predicted
NNMT	Nicotinamide N-methyltransferase (ENSG00000166741)	Predicted
NOS1AP	Nitric oxide synthase 1 (neuronal) adaptor protein (ENSG00000198929)	Predicted
NUFIP1	Nuclear fragile X mental retardation protein interacting protein 1 (ENSG00000083635)	Predicted
PEX1	Peroxisomal biogenesis factor 1 (ENSG00000127980)	Predicted
PLSCR1	Phospholipid scramblase 1 (ENSG00000188313)	Predicted
PPM1B	Protein phosphatase, Mg2+/Mn2+ dependent, 1B (ENSG00000138032)	Predicted
PPP4R1L	Protein phosphatase 4, regulatory subunit 1-like (ENSG00000124224)	Predicted
PTHLH	Parathyroid hormone-like hormone (ENSG00000087494)	Predicted

Table 5.3—(*continued*)

Gene	Description	Evidence
SCP2	Sterol carrier protein 2 (ENSG00000116171)	Predicted
SLC16A7	Solute carrier family 16, member 7 (monocarboxylic acid transporter 2) (ENSG00000118596)	Predicted
SLC7A6OS	Solute carrier family 7, member 6 opposite strand (ENSG00000103061)	Predicted
ZNF274	Zinc finger protein 274 (ENSG00000171606)	Predicted
ZNF805	Zinc finger protein 805 (ENSG00000204524)	Predicted
ZFYVE28	Zinc finger, FYVE domain containing 28 (ENSG00000159733)	Predicted

Sources: miRSearch www.mirdb.org, and www.mirbase.org. *Expression in progressors/nonprogressors.

Clearly, the association of specific miRNAs as well as entire miRNA profiles with disorders of glucose regulation, such as prediabetes and diabetes, makes these small molecules potentially useful plasma biomarkers and, hence, potential targets for novel therapeutic interventions.[21] Currently, information is incomplete on the genes regulated by differential microRNAs and how that translates to susceptibility to, or protection against, impaired glucose metabolism and development of prediabetes and diabetes.

References

1. Bartel DP. MicroRNAs: genomics, biogenesis, mechanism, and function. *Cell* 2004;116:281
2. Ross JS, Carlson JA, Brock G. miRNA: the new gene silencer. *Am J Clin Path* 2007;128:830–836
3. Ghildiyal M, Zamore PD. Small silencing RNAs: an expanding universe. *Nat Rev Genet* 2009;10:94–108
4. Friedman RC, Farh KK, Burge CB, Bartel DP. Most mammalian mRNAs are conserved targets of microRNAs. *Genome Res* 2009;19:92–105
5. Chien HY, Lee TP, Chen CY, et al. Circulating microRNA as a diagnostic marker in populations with type 2 diabetes mellitus and diabetic complications. *J Chin Med Assoc* 2015;78:204–211
6. Shantikumar S, Caporali A, Emanueli C. Role of microRNAs in diabetes and its cardiovascular complications. *Cardiovas Res* 2012;93:583–593
7. Poy MN, Hausser J, Trajkovski M, et al. miR-375 maintains normal pancreatic alpha- and beta-cell mass. *Proc Natl Acad Sci U S A* 2009;106: 5813–5818

8. Xu G, Chen J, Jing G, Shalev A. Thioredoxin-interacting protein regulates insulin transcription through microRNA-204. *Nat Med* 2013;19: 1141–1146
9. Esguerra JL, Bolmeson C, Cilio CM, Eliasson L. Differential glucose-regulation of microRNAs in pancreatic islets of non-obese type 2 diabetes model Goto-Kakizaki rat. *PLoS One* 2011;6:e18613
10. Zhang T, Ji C, Shi R. miR-142-3p promotes pancreatic β cell survival through targeting FOXO1 in gestational diabetes mellitus. *Int J Clin Exp Pathol* 2019;12:1529–1538
11. Plaisance A, Waeber G, Regazzi R, Abderrahmani A. Role of microRNAs in islet beta-cell compensation and failure during diabetes. *J Diabetes Res* 2014;2014:618652
12. Assmann TS, Recamonde-Mendoza M, De Souza BM, Crispim D. MiroRNA expression profiles and type 1 diabetes mellitus: systematic review and bioinformatic analysis. *Endocr Connect* 2017;6:773–790
13. Zhu H, Leung SW. Identification of microRNA biomarkers in type 2 diabetes: a meta-analysis of controlled profiling studies. *Diabetologia* 2015;58:900–911
14. Zhang T, Lv C, Li L, et al. Plasma miR-126 is a potential biomarker for early prediction of type 2 diabetes mellitus in susceptible individuals. *Biomed Res Int* 2013:2013;761617
15. Sebastiani G, Po A, Miele E, et al. MicroRNA-124a is hyperexpressed in type diabetic human pancreatic islets and negatively regulates insulin secretion. *Acta Diabetol* 2015;52:523–530
16. Locke JM, da Silva Xavier G, Dawe HR, et al. Increased expression of miR-187 in human islets from individuals with type 2 diabetes is associated with reduced glucose-stimulated insulin secretion. *Diabetologia* 2014;57:122–128
17. de Candia P, Spinetti G, Specchia C, et al. A unique plasma microRNA profile defines type 2 diabetes progression. *PLoS One* 2017;12:e0188980
18. Matsha TE, Kengne AP, Hector S, et al. MicroRNA profiling and their pathways in South African individuals with prediabetes and newly diagnosed type 2 diabetes mellitus. *Oncotarget* 2018;9:30485–30498
19. Owei I, Dokun AO, Stentz FB, Dagogo-Jack S. MicroRNA expression profiles and progression from normoglycemia to prediabetes in a biracial cohort. *Diabetes* 2020;69(Suppl. 1): https://doi.org/10.2337/db20-197-LB
20. Wang P, Liu Q, Zhao H, et al. miR-216a-targeting theranostic nanoparticles promote proliferation of insulin-secreting cells in type 1 diabetes animal model. *Sci Rep* 2020;10:5302
21. Kim M, Zhang X. The profiling and role of miRNAs in diabetes mellitus. *J Diabetes Clin Res* 2019;1:5–23

Metabolomics and Prediabetes

The science of metabolomics involves the assessment of circulating concentrations of small molecules and metabolites in relation to their impact on integrated metabolic pathophysiology, particularly with respect to the regulation of carbohydrate and lipid metabolism and overall cardiometabolic health.[1–3] The small molecules and metabolites include branched-chain amino acids (BCAAs) (isoleucine, leucine, and valine) and aromatic amino acids (AAAs) (phenylalanine, tyrosine), along with methionine, glutamine, acylcarnitines, urea cycle intermediates, purine degradation products, bile acids, ketone bodies, and lipid moieties.[1–3] The circulating levels of these metabolites are typically assayed with liquid chromatography/mass spectrometry. Pioneering studies in the predominantly white Framingham Heart Study Offspring cohort documented robust associations between baseline levels of BCAAs and two AAAs and the risk of incident type 2 diabetes after 12 years of follow-up.[4] Those associations were replicated in another white cohort, the Malmö Diet and Cancer study.[4] Several subsequent reports have linked alterations in plasma levels of certain amino acids and the risk of type 2 diabetes in diverse populations, but the specific metabolites and direction of association have been variable.[5–9]

In the Framingham Heart Study, elevated baseline levels of three BCAAs (isoleucine, leucine, and valine) and two AAAs (tyrosine and phenylalanine) among initially normoglycemic individuals strongly predicted future risk of type 2 diabetes.[4] As reported, the combination of any three of these five amino acids improved the prediction of future diabetes, compared with individual amino acids. Notably, the combination of isoleucine, phenylalanine, and tyrosine showed the strongest predictive power for future type 2 diabetes: individuals at the top quartile of that trio of amino acids had a greater than five-fold increased risk of future diabetes, compared to individuals in the lowest quartile.[4] However, among participants in the multiethnic Insulin Resistance Atherosclerosis Study, the signature that predicted increased future risk of type 2 diabetes was characterized by decreased glycine, and increased valine, leucine, phenylalanine, and glutamine/glutamate levels, at baseline.[5] In another multiethnic cohort, the Diabetes Prevention Program, which tracked progression to type 2 diabetes among participants with prediabetes, a different profile (lower baseline levels of glycine betaine and serine, and higher levels of methionine sulfoxide, and propionylcarnitine) was found to significantly predict incident type 2 diabetes, after adjustments for multiple baseline variables.[6] The previously reported diabetes risk predictors (BCAAs and AAAs) did not emerge as significant predictors in the Diabetes Prevention Program cohort, after adjustment for baseline variables, including age, sex, race/ethnicity, BMI, and fasting plasma glucose levels.[6] Thus, it appears that the pattern of amino acids associated with type 2 diabetes may differ based on the race/ethnic background of the population studied.

In addition to the numerous reports of associations between amino acid profiles and incident type 2 diabetes, some studies have examined the role of amino acids in prediabetes.[10–13] Using a nontargeted metabolomics approach, in which 447 fasting plasma metabolites were assayed in a cross-sectional comparison of 192 individuals with prediabetes (impaired fasting glucose) and 1,897 healthy control subjects, Menni et al.[10] identified 14 metabolites that were associated with impaired fasting glucose. Among the latter, 3-methyl-2-oxovalerate (a branched-chain keto acid metabolite) showed the strongest association with prediabetes, with an OR of 1.65 (95% CI 1.39–1.95). The OR in relation to prediabetes was 1.55 (1.29–1.86) for isoleucine, 1.46 (1.21–1.76) for leucine, and 1.36 (1.14–1.62) for valine.[10] In another cross-sectional study, the plasma levels of five BCAAs (isoleucine, leucine, valine, phenylalanine, and tyrosine) were analyzed in 898 patients with hypertension (171 with comorbid prediabetes [impaired fasting glucose] and 727 with normoglycemia).[11] The authors found weak associations between impaired fasting glucose and each of the five BCAAs among European American subjects (adjusted ORs of 1.007–1.031 per μmol/L increase in level), but only valine was associated with impaired fasting glucose among African American participants.[11] In other reports, lower levels of glycine have been associated with increased risk of prevalent prediabetes.[12]

A major limitation of these cross-sectional studies is that they do not permit inferences as to whether the observed amino acid patterns preceded the development of prediabetes, or resulted from the dysmetabolic milieu associated with the prediabetic state. Prospective studies are needed to address that quandary. In the only prospective study reported to date, Owei et al.[13] analyzed whether the three BCAAs (isoleucine, leucine, and valine) and two AAAs (tyrosine and phenylalanine), known to predict type 2 diabetes risk, were also significant predictors of prediabetes risk in a population of African Americans and European Americans. The study subjects who were participants in the POP-ABC study enrolled with normoglycemia and were followed up for progression to incident prediabetes over a period of 5.5 years.[13] Using a case-control study design, Owei et al.[13] compared baseline plasma levels of 18 amino acids in progressors to prediabetes ($N = 70$) and nonprogressors ($N = 70$). The two groups were matched for age, sex, and ethnicity. Table 5.4 shows the list of 18 amino acids and their mean concentrations in fasting plasma samples obtained at baseline. The total plasma level of amino acids correlated significantly with lean mass ($r = 0.36$, $P < 0.0001$), waist circumference ($r = 0.27$, $P = 0.001$), fasting plasma glucose ($r = 0.24$, $P = 0.005$), homeostasis model assessment–insulin resistance (HOMA-IR) ($r = 0.22$, $P = 0.01$), and HDL cholesterol level ($r = -0.18$, $P = 0.03$). The authors found that plasma levels of 12 of the 18 amino acids did not differ significantly in progressors and nonprogressors, whereas the levels of six amino acids (glutamic acid, glutamine, histidine, phenylalanine, aspartic acid, and asparagine) were discordant between the two groups.

Table 5.4—Comparison of Fasting Plasma Amino Acid Levels (µmol/L) in Progressors to Prediabetes and Nonprogressors[13]

	Progressors	Nonprogressors	*P*
Total amino acids	1,730 ± 194	1,687 ± 195	0.20
Alanine	335 ± 81.2	335 ± 71.2	0.99
Arginine	83.0 ± 19.8	77.5 ± 18.7	0.10
Aspartic acid + asparagine	14.2 ± 4.03	10.1 ± 3.91	<0.0001
Citrulline	29.8 ± 6.53	29.8 ± 6.33	0.99
Glutamic acid + glutamine	99.1 ± 19.1	90.0 ± 18.6	0.005
Glycine	261± 68.1	265 ± 74.6	0.73
Histidine	75.8 ± 7.94	79.8 ± 12.7	0.02
Isoleucine + leucine	154 ± 24.3	145 ± 29.9	0.07
Methionine	25.8 ± 4.02	25.8 ± 4.38	0.93
Ornithine	57.6 ± 13.2	54.3 ± 14.4	0.16
Phenylalanine	55.7 ± 7.13	52.9 ± 7.02	0.02
Proline	158 ± 37.1	155 ± 43.8	0.64
Serine	102 ± 18.2	99.2 ± 17.7	0.36
Tyrosine	61.3 ± 11.2	58.4 ± 12.6	0.15
Valine	218 ± 34.7	208 ± 41.8	0.17

Leucine and isoleucine, being isobaric, appeared together at the same mass, and their levels were combined. During hot, acidic esterification, some or all asparagine molecules were converted to aspartic acid, so the combined asparagine and aspartate concentration was reported. Similarly, glutamine molecules are converted to glutamic acid during hot, acidic esterification; their combined concentration was reported.

After adjustment for age, sex, race, and BMI, the only significant amino acids predictive of incident prediabetes were the combined mass of aspartic acid plus asparagine and histidine.[13] (During the acidic esterification step of sample preparation, some or all asparagine molecules are converted to aspartic acid, so the analysis combined asparagine and aspartate concentrations.) Each 1-SD increase in baseline aspartic acid plus asparagine levels predicted a 2.72-fold higher risk of incident prediabetes, whereas a 1-SD increase in baseline histidine levels predicted a 10% lower risk of incident prediabetes.[13] The OR for prediabetes risk associated with histidine was 0.92 (95% CI 0.86–0.98, $P = 0.00118$) in African American participants and 0.85 (0.75–0.97, $P = 0.0133$) in European American subjects. The OR for increased prediabetes risk associated with aspartic acid plus asparagine was four-fold greater in European American subjects (9.57 [95% CI 2.56–35.7], $P = 0.0008$) compared with African American subjects (2.05 [95% CI 1.41–2.98], $P = 0.0002$). The BCAAs (isoleucine, leucine, and valine) and the AAA tyrosine did not significantly predict incident prediabetes in the POP-ABC study. Thus, the amino acid signature predictive of incident prediabetes in a prospective biracial cohort was quite different from that reported for incident type 2 diabetes in the predominantly white Framingham Offspring cohort.[4,13]

The mechanisms linking higher levels of certain amino acids to increased risk of dysglycemia are not fully understood. Circulating amino acid levels reflect a balance among dietary intake, protein synthesis, proteolysis, and catabolism of excess amino acids. Hyperaminoacidemia thus indicates either overproduction (diet delivery and proteolysis) or impaired clearance (use in protein synthesis, catabolism, and conversion to Kreb's cycle intermediates). Because insulin stimulates protein synthesis and inhibits proteolysis, states of insulin deficiency or insulin resistance could lead to hyperaminoacidemia. Furthermore, insulin-resistant states are associated with decreased activity of key enzymes involved in the catabolism of BCAAs.[14] Thus, mechanisms of elevated fasting plasma levels of BCAAs and other amino acids include insulin resistance, relative insulin deficiency, or decreased amino acid catabolism, all of which can induce glucose dysregulation. Additionally, circulating BCAAs and other amino acids can induce insulin resistance via activation of the molecular target of rapamycin (mTOR), AMPK, and other pathways.[15] Underscoring the significance of the link between BCAAs and type 2 diabetes is the observation that gastric bypass surgery, which rapidly improves glucose tolerance (independently of weight loss), significantly decreases plasma BCAA levels.[16] In the latter report, metabolomic profiles were compared before and after a matched 10-kg weight loss induced by gastric bypass or diet: total amino acids, BCAAs, and metabolites derived from BCAA oxidation all decreased after gastric bypass, but not after dietary intervention.[16] The decrease in circulating amino acids after gastric bypass was associated with improved insulin sensitivity. Given the identical weight loss in both groups, the decrease is likely mediated by mechanisms other than weight loss.[16] The proposed mechanisms of the decrease in plasma amino acids after gastric bypass include decreased protein intake, increased catabolism, and/or decreased protein degradation.[16]

The finding that higher histidine levels predicted a lower risk of incident prediabetes is probably explained by the well-documented beneficial effects of histidine in ameliorating or reversing systemic and adipose tissue inflammation, oxidative stress, adiposity, and ingestive behavior.[17–19] In additional mechanistic studies, Owei et al.[13] demonstrated significant associations between individual plasma amino acid levels and insulin sensitivity and insulin secretion. Interestingly, the hydrophobic amino acid glycine showed a positive association with insulin sensitivity and an inverse association with insulin secretion, whereas the AAAs (phenylalanine and tyrosine) and polar amino acids (glutamine and glutamic acid) were inversely associated with insulin sensitivity and positively associated with insulin secretion (Fig. 5.2). The observation regarding glycine is in accord with

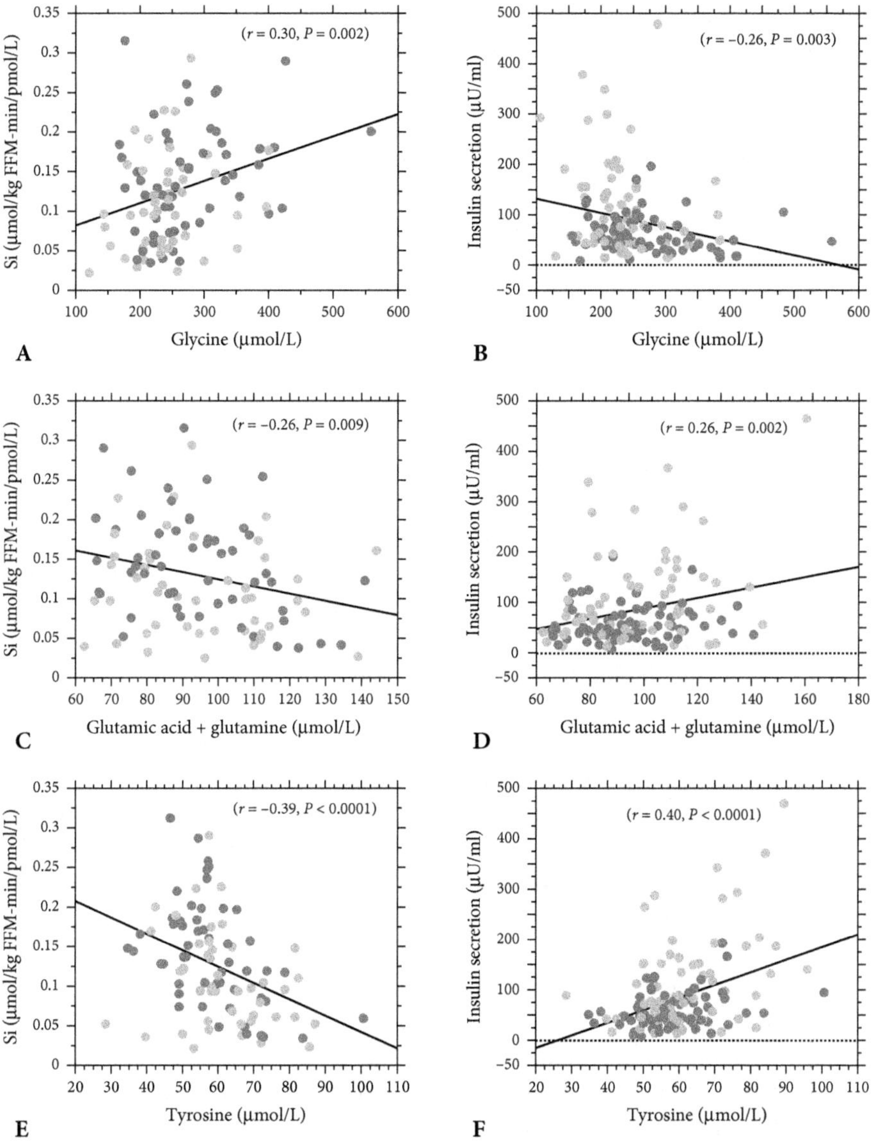

Figure 5.2—Association of fasting plasma levels of glycine (*A* and *B*), glutamic acid and glutamine (*C* and *D*), and tyrosine (*E* and *F*) with insulin sensitivity (Si) (upper panels) and insulin secretion (lower panels) in normoglycemic African American subjects (blue circles) and European American subjects (red circles).[13] FFM, fat-free mass.

reports of beneficial association between higher glycine levels and decreased cardiometabolic risk.[20–23] Glycine, a nonessential amino acid and a precursor for creatinine, purine, and collagen synthesis, has been associated with anti-inflammatory, immunomodulatory, and antioxidant properties.[20–23] Glycine receptors are expressed on pancreatic β-cells (21), and dietary glycine supplementation improves antioxidant and metabolic functions.[22,23] Thus, the emerging science of metabolomics could inspire the design of targeted dietary or nutraceutical approaches based on selective exclusion of unfavorable metabolites and selective enrichment with pro-metabolic nutrients.

References

1. Dagogo-Jack S. Metabolomic prediction of diabetes and cardiovascular risk. *Med Princ Pract* 2012;21:401–403
2. Newgard CB, An J, Bain JR, et al. A branched-chain amino acid-related metabolic signature that differentiates obese and lean humans and contributes to insulin resistance. *Cell Metab* 2009;9:311–326
3. Huffman KM, Shah SH, Stevens RD, et al. Relationships between circulating metabolic intermediates and insulin action in overweight to obese, inactive men and women. *Diabetes Care* 2009;32:1678–1683
4. Wang TJ, Larson MG, Vasan RS, et al. Metabolite profiles and the risk of developing diabetes. *Nat Med* 2011;17:448–453
5. Palmer ND, Stevens RD, Antinozzi PA, et al. Metabolomic profile associated with insulin resistance and conversion to diabetes in the Insulin Resistance Atherosclerosis Study. *J Clin Endocrinol Metab* 2015;100: E463–E468
6. Walford GA, Ma Y, Clish C, et al.; Diabetes Prevention Program Research Group. Metabolite profiles of diabetes incidence and intervention response in the Diabetes Prevention Program. *Diabetes* 2016;65:1424–1433
7. Jainandunsing S, Wattimena JL, Verhoeven AJ, et al. Discriminative ability of plasma branched-chain amino acid levels for glucose intolerance in families at risk for type 2 diabetes. *Metab Syndr Relat Disord* 2016;14: 175–181
8. van Valkengoed IGM, Argmann C, Ghauharali-van der Vlugt K, et al. Ethnic differences in metabolite signatures and type 2 diabetes: a nested case-control analysis among people of South Asian, African and European origin. *Nutr Diabetes* 2017;7:300
9. Cheng S, Rhee EP, Larson MG, et al. Metabolite profiling identifies pathways associated with metabolic risk in humans. *Circulation* 2012;125: 2222–2231

10. Menni C, Fauman E, Erte I, et al. Biomarkers for type 2 diabetes and impaired fasting glucose using a non-targeted metabolomics approach. *Diabetes* 2013;62:4270–4276
11. Weng L, Quinlivan E, Gong Y, et al. Association of branched and aromatic amino acids levels with metabolic syndrome and impaired fasting glucose in hypertensive patients. *Metab Syndr Relat Disord* 2015;13:195–202
12. Gar C, Rottenkolber M, Prehn C, et al. Serum and plasma amino acids as markers of prediabetes, insulin resistance, and incident diabetes. *Crit Rev Clin Lab Sci* 2018;55:21–32
13. Owei I, Umekwe U, Stentz F, et al. Amino acid signature predictive of incident prediabetes: a case-control study nested within the longitudinal Pathobiology of Prediabetes in a Biracial Cohort Metabolism. *Metabolism* 2019;98:76–83
14. She P, Van Horn C, Reid T, et al. Obesity related elevations in plasma leucine are associated with alterations in enzymes involved in branched-chain amino acid metabolism. *Am J Physiol Endocrinol Metab* 2007;293:E1552–E1563
15. Lu J, Xie G, Jia W, Jia W. Insulin resistance and the metabolism of branched-chain amino acids. *Front Med* 2013;7:53–59
16. Laferrère B, Reilly D, Arias S, et al. Differential metabolic impact of gastric bypass surgery versus dietary intervention in obese diabetic subjects despite identical weight loss. *Sci Transl Med* 2011;3:80re2
17. Feng RN, Niu YC, Sun XW, et al. Histidine supplementation improves insulin resistance through suppressed inflammation in obese women with the metabolic syndrome: a randomised controlled trial. *Diabetologia* 2013;56:985–994
18. Kasaoka S, Tsuboyama-Kasaoka N, Kawahara Y, et al. Histidine supplementation suppresses food intake and fat accumulation in rats. *Nutrition* 2004;20:991–996
19. DiNicolantonio JJ, McCarty MF, OKeefe JH. Role of dietary histidine in the prevention of obesity and metabolic syndrome. *Open Heart* 2018;5:e000676
20. Razak MA, Begum PS, Viswanath B, Rajagopal S. Multifarious beneficial effect of non-essential amino acid, glycine: a review. *Oxid Med Cell Longev* 2017;2017;1716701
21. Yan-Do R, Duong E, Manning Fox JE, et al. A glycine-insulin autocrine feedback loop enhances insulin secretion from human β-cells and is impaired in type 2 diabetes. *Diabetes* 2016;65:2311–2321
22. Gannon MC, Nuttall JA, Nuttall FQ. The metabolic response to ingested glycine. *Am J Clin Nutr* 2002;76:1302–1307
23. Sekhar RV, McKay SV, Patel SG, et al. Glutathione synthesis is diminished in patients with uncontrolled diabetes and restored by dietary supplementation with cysteine and glycine. *Diabetes Care* 2011;34:162–167

Acylcarnitines Levels in Prediabetes

Dietary lipids are absorbed as fatty acids and esterified in the cytosol to long-chain fatty acyl-CoA. The long-chain acyl-CoAs are shepherded into mitochondria via the carnitine shuttle, during which the long-chain acyl-CoAs are converted to acylcarnitines by carnitine palmitoyltransferase (CPT)-1 located in the outer mitochondrial membrane.[1–3] Next, the mitochondrial inner membrane transporter carnitine acylcarnitine translocase (CACT or SLC25A20) delivers the acylcarnitines into the mitochondrial matrix.[1–3] From there, the enzyme CPT-2 reconverts acylcarnitines back into long-chain acyl-CoAs for oxidation and free carnitine.[1–3] Acylcarnitines can be measured in plasma, indicating their efflux from mitochondria. It has been suggested that circulating acylcarnitine levels reflect mitochondrial overload and incomplete fatty acid oxidation.[4] Higher plasma levels of certain acylcarnitines have been reported in insulin-resistant states, such as obesity and type 2 diabetes.[5–8]

Zhang et al.[9] measured serum acylcarnitines in 61 adults (mean age 51 years), of whom 20 were normal glucose tolerant, 20 had prediabetes, and 21 had newly diagnosed type 2 diabetes. Compared with the normal glucose tolerant control subjects, individuals with type 2 diabetes and prediabetes had significantly higher levels of long-chain acylycarnithines: palmitoylcarnitine (C16), 3-OH-hexadecanoylcarnitine (C16-OH), carnitine C20, carnitine C22, and carnitine C24. The higher levels of the long-chain acylcarnitines were evident when comparing subjects with normal glucose tolerance or prediabetes with type 2 diabetes subjects, but the levels were somewhat similar between subjects with prediabetes and subjects with type 2 diabetes.[9] No differences were noted in the levels of short- and medium-chain acylcarnitines.[9] Another cross-sectional study compared plasma levels of 24 acylcarnitines in 1,019 subjects, including 635 with normal glucose tolerance, 271 with prediabetes (184 with impaired fasting glucose and 87 with impaired glucose tolerance), and 112 with type 2 diabetes.[10] The analysis showed differences in short-, medium-, and long-chain acylcarnitines across the glycemic groups.[10] Within the prediabetes group, the levels of C14:1, C14:2, and C18:1 were reported to be significantly higher in individuals with impaired glucose tolerance than in individuals with impaired fasting glucose.[10] The authors also noted that the impaired fasting glucose and impaired glucose tolerance subjects showed lower serum concentrations of malonylcarnitine/hydroxybutyrylcarnitine (C3DC+C4OH) than the type 2 diabetes group.[10]

These cross-sectional observations indicate that dysregulation in fat oxidation, as indicated by acylcarnitine levels, precedes the occurrence of diabetes and is evident at the stage of prediabetes. However, determining whether the dysregulation precedes or follows the development of prediabetes requires prospective studies. In that regard, baseline plasma levels of 45 acylcarnitines were analyzed and

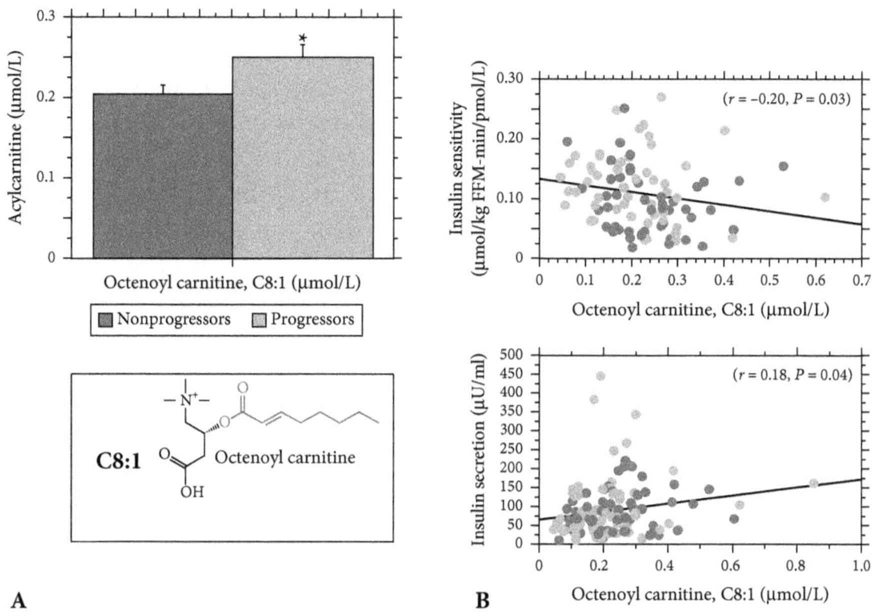

Figure 5.3—*A*: Comparison of plasma levels of C8:1 subjects who progressed from normoglycemia to prediabetes (progressors) or maintained normoglycemia (nonprogressors) during 5.5 years of follow-up in the POP-ABC study. *B*: Association of C8:1 levels with insulin sensitivity and insulin secretion in African Americans (blue circles) and European Americans (red circles).[10] **P* = 0.01.

compared among initially normoglycemic participants in the POP-ABC study who developed incident prediabetes (progressors, $N = 70$) during the 5.5-year follow-up and 70 age-, sex-, and ethnicity-matched control subjects who maintained normoglycemia during follow-up (nonprogressors).[11] Of the 45 acylcarnitines analyzed, progressors and nonprogressors were concordant for 36 and discordant for 9. Compared to nonprogressors, the progressors had higher baseline levels of C8:1 (octenoyl carnitine), but lower levels of C4-OH (β-hydroxy butyryl carnitine), C4-DC/Ci4-DC (methylmalonyl carnitine/succinyl carnitine), C5-DC (glutaryl carnitine), C5-OH/C3-DC (3-hydroxy-isovaleryl carnitine/ malonyl carnitine), C14 (myristoyl carnitine), C16 (palmitoyl carnitine), C18 (stearoyl carnitine), and C18:2 (linoleoyl carnitine) (Table 5.3, Fig. 5.3). Plasma levels of C8:1 (octenoyl carnitine) correlated inversely with insulin sensitivity, which suggests it might be a marker of insulin resistance (Fig. 5.3). Thus, the higher levels of C8:1 observed in progressors to prediabetes seem pathophysiologically congruent. In a multivariate regression model, including all nine discordant acylcarnitines, C4-OH ($P = 0.002$) and C8:1 ($P = 0.005$) emerged as the strongest significant predictors of incident prediabetes.[11]

Thus, in a prospective study of acylcarnitines and glucoregulation in a biracial cohort of initially normoglycemic subjects, baseline plasma levels of several short- and long-chain acylcarnitines were associated with insulin sensitivity and predicted the risk of incident prediabetes. The association was strongest for C4-OH and C8:1. These data indicate that impaired fatty acid oxidation, as indicated by circulating acylcarnitines, indeed precedes the development of prediabetes. Based on this finding, certain acylcarnitines may emerge as sensitive biomarkers and predictors of early glucose abnormalities.

References

1. Eaton S. Control of mitochondrial beta-oxidation flux. *Prog Lipid Res* 2002;41:197–239
2. Rasmussen BB, Holmbäck UC, Volpi E, et al. Malonyl coenzyme A and the regulation of functional carnitine palmitoyltransferase-1 activity and fat oxidation in human skeletal muscle. *J Clin Invest* 2002;110:1687–1693
3. Ramsay RR, Gandour RD, van der Leij FR. Molecular enzymology of carnitine transfer and transport. *Biochim Biophys Acta* 2001;1546:21–43
4. Koves TR, Ussher JR, Noland RC, et al. Mitochondrial overload and incomplete fatty acid oxidation contribute to skeletal muscle insulin resistance. *Cell Metab* 2008;7:45–56
5. Muoio DM, Neufer PD. Lipid-induced mitochondrial stress and insulin action in muscle. *Cell Metab* 2012;15:595–605
6. Mihalik SJ, Goodpaster BH, Kelley DE, et al. Increased levels of plasma acylcarnitines in obesity and type 2 diabetes and identification of a marker of glucolipotoxicity. *Obesity (Silver Spring)* 2010;18:1695–1700
7. Schooneman MG, Vaz FM, Houten SM, Soeters MR. Acylcarnitines: reflecting or inflicting insulin resistance? *Diabetes* 2013;62:1–8
8. Morino K, Petersen KF, Shulman GI. Molecular mechanisms of insulin resistance in humans and their potential links with mitochondrial dysfunction. *Diabetes* 2006;55(Suppl. 2):S9–S15
9. Zhang X, Zhang C, Chen L, et al. Human serum acylcarnitine profiles in different glucose tolerance states. *Diabetes Res Clin Pract* 2014;104:376–382
10. Mai M, Tönjes A, Kovacs P, et al. Serum levels of acylcarnitines are altered in prediabetic conditions. *PLoS One* 2013;8:e82459
11. Owei I, Umekwe N, Stentz F, Wan J, Dagogo-Jack S. Association of plasma acylcarnitines with insulin sensitivity, insulin secretion, and prediabetes in a biracial cohort. *Exp Biol Med* 2021 Epub April 29, 2021 https://journals.sagepub.com/doi/10.1177/15353702211009493

The Gut Microbiome in Prediabetes

There is a growing understanding from studies in rodents and humans that gut flora and the metagenome, rather than being passive commensals, may be actively involved in host-signaling pathways that can influence cardiometabolic health and susceptibility to obesity and diabetes.[1–5] Cross-sectional studies of age-, sex-, and BMI-matched subjects with or without diabetes have shown compositional changes in the gut microbiota that are associated with diabetes.[6,7] Differences in gut flora have also been described when comparing individuals with normal glucose tolerance, prediabetes, or newly diagnosed type 2 diabetes.[8] Individuals with prediabetes or type 2 diabetes were reported to have a lower abundance of Verrucomicrobiae compared to the normal glucose tolerance group.[8] A pattern characterized by higher abundance of Anaerostipes and lower abundances of Ruminococcaceae and Christensenellaceae was reported among middle-aged Finnish men with prediabetes.[9] Larger, metagenome-wide association studies have shown that type 2 diabetes is associated with decreased abundance of butyrate-producing bacteria and increased abundance of other species.[10,11] Karlsson et al.[11] applied a metagenome-wide approach to distinguish patterns of gut flora in European women with normal glucose tolerance, impaired glucose tolerance, and type 2 diabetes in cross-sectional comparisons.

Thus, the evidence is accumulating showing that gut microbiota interact with host metabolic pathways in ways that could influence susceptibility to prediabetes and diabetes. The interaction between gut flora and host metabolic function may be mediated, at least in part, by the effects of those flora on the availability of AAAs and BCAAs. Gut bacteria extract amino acids from dietary protein or other endogenous sources in the host and use the amino acids for protein synthesis. Alimentary bacteria also are sources of several essential amino acids derived from microbial synthesis or protein catabolism.[12,13] As discussed in the preceding section, circulating levels of certain amino acids (including BCAAs and AAAs) have been associated with insulin resistance, prediabetes, and type 2 diabetes.

The microbiome field is still in a state of flux, and the profiles of microbiota dysbiosis associated with diabetes or prediabetes tend to differ by age, geographical location, ethnic origin of the study population, and specific techniques. Prospective studies are needed to dissect out the specific role of gut flora and the metagenome during transition from normal glucose regulation to prediabetes and subsequent development of type 2 diabetes. Such foundational studies could lead to novel insights regarding the possibility of manipulating gut flora as a strategy for prevention of prediabetes and type 2 diabetes.[14] Such knowledge could also identify environmental exposures that might increase the risks of obesity, prediabetes, and diabetes via unfavorable alteration of gut flora.[15,16] For example, a nested case-control study from the Health Improvement Network (a large population-based database in the United Kingdom) indicated that exposure to two to five courses of antibiotics (≥1 year before the index date) was associated with an increased risk of incident diabetes during ~18 years of follow-up.[16] Specifically, the adjusted OR (95% CI) for treatment with penicillin, cephalosporins, macrolides, and quinolones ranged from 1.08 (95% CI 1.05–1.11) for penicillin to 1.15 (95% CI 1.08–1.23) for quinolones. The diabetes risk increased with the number of antibiotic courses, reaching 1.37 (95% CI 1.19–1.58) for more than five courses of quinolones.[16] No association was observed between diabetes risk and treatment with anti-viral and anti-fungal agents.[16]

The relationship between antibiotic exposure and incident diabetes persisted after adjusting for BMI, smoking, prestudy glucose level, number of infections, and other pertinent factors.[16] Although no conclusions regarding causality can be inferred from this retrospective case-control study, the results do implicate frequent use of certain antibiotics as possibly posing a risk for diabetes, presumably via effects on gut flora. Greater insight from future studies could potentially identify probiotics or other interventions that can counteract the presumed antibiotic-associated gut microbial dysbiosis leading to increased diabetes risk.

References

1. Turnbaugh PJ, Ley RE, Mahowald MA, et al. An obesity-associated gut microbiome with increased capacity for energy harvest. *Nature* 2006;444:1027–1031
2. Turnbaugh PJ, Hamady M, Yatsunenko T, et al. A core gut microbiome in obese and lean twins. *Nature* 2009;457:480–484
3. Ridaura VK, Faith JJ, Rey FE, et al. Gut microbiota from twins discordant for obesity modulate metabolism in mice. *Science* 2013;341:1241214
4. Koeth RA, Wang Z, Levison BS, et al. Intestinal microbiota metabolism of L-carnitine, a nutrient in red meat, promotes atherosclerosis. *Nat Med* 2013;19:576–585
5. Vrieze A, Van Nood E, Holleman F, et al. Transfer of intestinal microbiota from lean donors increases insulin sensitivity in individuals with metabolic syndrome. *Gastroenterology* 2012;143:913–916
6. Tai N, Wong FS, Wen L. The role of gut microbiota in the development of type 1, type 2 diabetes mellitus and obesity. *Rev Endocr Metab Disord* 2015;16:55–65
7. Moreno-Indias I, Cardona F, Tinahones FJ, Queipo-Ortuño MI. Impact of the gut microbiota on the development of obesity and type 2 diabetes mellitus. *Front Microbiol* 2014;5:190

8. Zhang X, Shen D, Fang Z, et al. Human gut microbiota changes reveal the progression of glucose intolerance. *PLoS One* 2013;8:e71108
9. Org E, Blum Y, Kasela S, et al. Relationships between gut microbiota, plasma metabolites, and metabolic syndrome traits in the METSIM cohort. *Genome Biol* 2017;18:70
10. Qin J, Li Y, Cai Z, et al. A metagenome-wide association study of gut microbiota in type 2 diabetes. *Nature* 2012;490:55–60
11. Karlsson FH, Tremaroli V, Nookaew I, et al. Gut metagenome in European women with normal, impaired and diabetic glucose control. *Nature* 2013;498:99–103
12. Neis EP, Dejong CH, Rensen SS. The role of microbial amino acid metabolism in host metabolism. *Nutrients* 2015;7:2930–2946
13. Lin R, Liu W, Piao M, Zhu H. A review of the relationship between the gut microbiota and amino acid metabolism. *Amino Acids* 2017;49: 2083–2090
14. Million M, Raoult D. The role of the manipulation of the gut microbiota in obesity. *Curr Infect Dis Rep* 2013;15:25–30
15. Azad MB, Bridgman SL, Becker AB, Kozyrskyj AL. Infant antibiotic exposure and the development of childhood overweight and central adiposity. *Int J Obes (Lond)* 2014;38:1290–1298
16. Boursi B, Mamtani R, Haynes K, Yang YX. The effect of past antibiotic exposure on diabetes risk. *Eur J Endocrinol* 2015;172:639–648

Chapter 6

Sequelae of Prediabetes: Progression to Type 2 Diabetes and Development of Premature Microvascular and Macrovascular Complications

Predictors of Progression from Prediabetes to Type 2 Diabetes

Individuals with prediabetes far outnumber those with diabetes. Estimates by the Centers for Disease Control and Prevention in the United States indicate that there are 34.2 million adults with diabetes and 88 million with prediabetes.[1] Individuals with prediabetes are the primary source of future cases of type 2 diabetes. An analysis of six prospective studies[2] on progression from prediabetes (impaired glucose tolerance) to type 2 diabetes identified the following features: *1*) higher baseline fasting plasma glucose and the 2-h oral glucose tolerance test glucose values predicted increased risk of progression to type 2 diabetes; *2*) the rate of progression from impaired glucose tolerance to type 2 diabetes was exponential among individuals in the top quartile of baseline fasting plasma glucose; *3*) incident diabetes rates displayed ethnic disparities, with higher rates occurring in Hispanics, Native Americans, and Nauruan populations than in whites; *4*) the degree of obesity predicted diabetes risk among study populations with low incidence rates of diabetes, but not in the studies that recorded the highest incidence of diabetes; and *5*) a family history of diabetes was a variable predictor of progression from impaired glucose tolerance to diabetes, suggesting that genetic effects probably are fully established by stage of impaired glucose tolerance in some individuals.[2] A population-based prospective study in England that stratified participants by baseline fasting glucose status showed that the 10-year incidence of type 2 diabetes per 1,000 person-years was 2.4 in individuals with normoglycemia (fasting plasma glucose <5.5 mmol/L or <100 mg/dL), 6.2 in individuals whose fasting plasma glucose was 5.6–6.0 mmol/L (100–109 mg/dL), and 17.5 in individuals whose fasting plasma glucose was 6.1–6.9 mmol/L (110–125 mg/dL).[3] Thus, the magnitude of fasting and post-challenge glycemia (indicative of insulin resistance and impaired insulin secretion) along with weight gain are important predictors of progression to type 2 diabetes.

Weight gain

Longitudinal studies in a high-risk population (Pima Indians) with baseline normal glucose tolerance indicated that weight gain, insulin resistance, and progressive loss of insulin secretory function are significant predictors of incident type 2 diabetes.[4] Weight gain predicted progression from normal glucose tolerance to impaired glucose tolerance (5.2 vs. 2.6 kg in nonprogressors); progression from impaired glucose tolerance to type 2 diabetes was associated with an additional weight gain of 13 kg (vs. 6 kg in nonprogressors) over a 5-year follow-up period.[4] The greater weight gain in the progressors was associated with an ~30% decline in insulin sensitivity and >50% decline in acute insulin secretory response to intravenous glucose.[4] Weight gain also predicted future development of type 2 diabetes among African American participants in the Atherosclerosis Risk in Communities study.[5] Thus, interventions that induce weight loss or prevented further weight gain could prevent progression from prediabetes to type 2 diabetes.

Insulin resistance

Impaired insulin-stimulated glucose transport into tissues (insulin resistance) was documented in first-degree relatives (with either normal glucose tolerance or impaired glucose tolerance) of individuals with type 2 diabetes.[6–8] Defective non-oxidative glucose disposal in skeletal muscles (i.e., glycogen synthesis) is a characteristic of insulin resistance.[7] In the Joslin Diabetes Center study,[8] insulin-resistant offspring of two parents with type 2 diabetes had an 80% increase in the risk of developing type 2 diabetes during a 25-year follow-up. Among Diabetes Prevention Program participants, progression from prediabetes to type 2 diabetes was inversely associated with baseline insulin sensitivity (hazard rate ratio 0.62–0.94 per SD difference, depending on assigned treatment group).[9] Together, these finding and other supportive data in the literature establish insulin resistance as a metabolic precursor to type 2 diabetes in different populations and provide a strong rationale for targeting insulin resistance as a strategy for diabetes prevention.

β-Cell dysfunction

In the prospective study of Pima Indians,[4] progressive decline in insulin secretion (evidence of β-cell dysfunction) was a critical determinant of progression from normal glucose tolerance to impaired glucose tolerance and from impaired glucose tolerance to type 2 diabetes. Evidence that β-cell dysfunction might be a heritable trait is provided by the observation of a high concordance rate for impaired insulin secretion among identical twins discordant for type 2 diabetes who were studied at an elderly age.[10] In the overall Diabetes Prevention Program cohort, all of whom had prediabetes at enrollment, the incidence of type 2 diabetes was significantly inversely related to baseline insulin secretion (hazard rate ratio 0.57–0.76 per SD).[9] The role of β-cell dysfunction in predicting progression to type 2 diabetes suggests that intervention that prevents the progressive decline in insulin secretion along with interventions that decrease insulin demand (by improving insulin sensitivity) can be expected to prevent or delay the development of type 2 diabetes.

The ultimate outcome of prediabetes in most people is either progression to type 2 diabetes or persistence in the prediabetes state. Spontaneous remission of prediabetes is a rare occurrence.[2,3] Indeed, after 30 years of follow-up of the participants in the Da Qing study (all of whom had prediabetes at enrollment), the cumulative incidence of type 2 diabetes was 95.9% in the control group and 88.7% in the diet and exercise intervention groups.[11] Similarly, after 15 years of follow-up of the Diabetes Prevention Program participants (all of whom had prediabetes at enrollment), the cumulative incidence of type 2 diabetes was 55% in the lifestyle group, 56% in the metformin group, and 62% in the placebo group.[12] Even in people who do not progress to type 2 diabetes, persistent prediabetes is a toxic state that is associated with increased risks for the initiation and progression of several microvascular and macrovascular complications.[13,14] The high likelihood of progression of type 2 diabetes along with the risk of premature vascular complications make prediabetes a serious diagnosis.[11–14] Arguments that prediabetes is a "dubious" diagnosis are ill-informed and cannot be further from the truth.[15]

Microvascular Complications of Prediabetes

The dogma has been that the development of microvascular complications of diabetes, namely retinopathy, neuropathy, and nephropathy, requires exposure to diabetes-grade hyperglycemia for several years or decades. However, the presence of these complications is being reported with increasing frequency in people with prediabetes[16–21] (Table 6.1). The occurrence of "long-term complications of diabetes" in some people with prediabetes is of grave public health concern, given the enormous size of the prediabetes population. In the Diabetes Prevention Program, 7.8% of subjects with impaired glucose tolerance had retinopathy,[19] close to the 8.1% prevalence of prediabetic retinopathy reported from the Gutenberg Health Study in Germany.[20] Microalbuminuria is seen in 15.5% of people with prediabetes.[20] Using an estimated glomerular filtrate rate, the presence of chronic kidney disease was documented in 17.7% of people with prediabetes in the National Health and Nutrition Examination Survey (NHANES) 1999–2006 cohort.[21] Classic

Table 6.1—Microvascular Complications of Prediabetes

Lesion	Prevalence	Population	Reference
Retinopathy	~8%	United States, Germany	16,17
Microalbuminuria	15.5%	Iran	18
Chronic kidney disease	17.7%	United States	19
Neuropathy	11–25%	United States, International	14,15

diabetic peripheral polyneuropathy (including painful episodes) was reported in 11–25% of individuals with prediabetes.[17,18] Among patients with idiopathic peripheral neuropathy, an estimated 25–62% have been reported to have prediabetes.[18] Manifestations of autonomic neuropathy, including reduced heart rate variability and erectile dysfunction, have been well documented in association with prediabetes.[17,18] These reports of premature occurrence of complications is buttressed by cognate findings of alterations in microvascular hemodynamics.[22,23]

The relationship between the duration of prediabetes and the development of microvascular complications cannot be determined, since these observations emanated from studies that enrolled people with prevalent prediabetes.[13–17] Thus, prospective studies of initially normoglycemic subjects followed up for incident prediabetes and then followed further for the occurrence of retinopathy (and other complications) in the prediabetes state would be required to determine the relationship.

Macrovascular Complications of Prediabetes

Beginning with the reports of the Paris Prospective Study that showed a doubling of cardiovascular disease mortality among people with impaired glucose tolerance compared to people with normal glucose tolerance, several studies observed increased risk of macrovascular complications in people with prediabetic blood glucose levels.[24–28] Increases in the risks of all the known macrovascular complications (coronary artery disease, myocardial infarction, congestive heart failure, stroke, peripheral vascular diseases, and cardiovascular disease death) have been reported in the prediabetes state compared with normoglycemia.[29] Among the ethnically diverse population enrolled in the Multi-Ethnic Study of Atherosclerosis (MESA), participants with prediabetes had a nearly three-fold higher prevalence of unrecognized myocardial infarction compared with their normoglycemic counterparts.[30] The association between prediabetes and increased risk of stroke extends to transient ischemic attack, recurrent stroke, and post-stroke prognosis as well.[31–34] Thus, similar to microvascular complications, there is well-documented evidence for increased risks of cardiovascular, cerebrovascular, and peripheral vascular complications in people with prediabetes.

Because people with prediabetes often harbor additional risk factors associated with the metabolic syndrome (insulin resistance, visceral adiposity, hypertension, dyslipidemia, and proinflammatory markers, among others), the increased macrovascular risk is likely not due to impaired glucose regulation alone. Nonetheless, epidemiological data from the EPIC-Norfolk study showed that a 1% increase in A1C, albeit within the normal range, was associated with an increased 10-year cardiovascular disease mortality.[28] The toxic role of the prediabetes state is underscored by findings that precursors to atherosclerosis, such as endothelial dysfunction, impaired endothelium-dependent vasodilation, vascular smooth muscle dysfunction, and increased arterial stiffness, have all been documented in people with prediabetes.[13,30,35,36] Similarly, whole-body MRI studies have revealed increased prevalence of subclinical cerebrovascular lesions (carotid plaque) and myocardial functional impairments (reduced early diastolic filling and late gadolinium enhancement) in people with prediabetes compared to normoglycemic control subjects.[37]

Interestingly, a randomized controlled study that targeted insulin resistance with pioglitazone in prediabetic patients (mean A1C 5.8 ± 0.4%) with a history of ischemic stroke or transient ischemic attack reported a significant decrease in the risks of recurrent stroke in the drug-treated group compared with the placebo control group. Along with decreased risk of stroke, the participants assigned to pioglitazone treatment also showed decreases in the rates of myocardial infarction and progression from prediabetes to type 2 diabetes.[38,39]

Mechanisms of prediabetic complications

Among people with established diabetes, some of the recognized mechanisms that contribute to microvascular complications include genetic predisposition; hyperglycemia-induced alterations in the polyol, hexosamine, and protein kinase C (PKC) pathways; advanced glycosylation end products; glomerular hyperfiltration; deleterious effects of growth factors; and inflammatory and oxidative stress, among others.[14,29,40] It is plausible that most of these processes may be operating at some level to drive premature microvascular complications in susceptible individuals with prediabetes, although direct mechanistic data are scant.

The role of hyperglycemia in the pathogenesis of microvascular complications is well established.[40] Elevated intracellular glucose levels activate toxic pathways (polyol pathway, advanced glycosylation end products, hexosamine pathway, and PKC activation) that mediate tissue damage (Fig. 6.1).[40] Based on conventional clinical experience, the tissue damage occurs after several years of exposure to uncontrolled hyperglycemia. Thus, it is unclear why some people with sub-diabetic glycemic levels become susceptible to the complications typically seen in patients

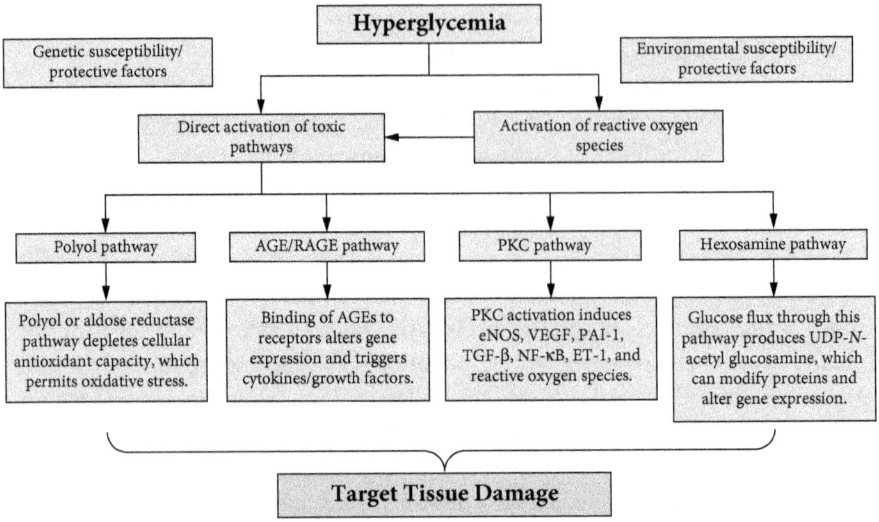

Figure 6.1—Intracellular pathways linking glucose to tissue damage.[38,39] AGE, advanced glycosylation end product; eNOS, endothelial nitric oxide synthase; ET-1, endothelin 1; NF-κB, nuclear factor-κB; PAI-1, plasminogen activator inhibitor-1; RAGE, receptor for AGE; TGF-β, transforming growth factor β; UDP, uridine diphosphate; VEGF, vascular endothelial growth factor.

with long-standing diabetes. One theoretical possibility is that there may be individual variability in the threshold of ambient glucose levels required for activation of toxic pathways.[14,29,40] Under that notion, genetic background and other putative co-factors could interact to render certain people susceptible to tissue damage at lower glucose exposure.[14,29] It is also conceivable that a multiplier effect could be in operation, whereby multiple toxic pathways[40] are activated in a manner that amplifies vulnerability to the development of premature microvascular and macrovascular complications in some people with prediabetes.[14,29,40]

Notably, activation of the PKC pathway by intracellular glucose unleashes a cascade of downstream mechanisms that amplify the toxicity of the initial glucose exposure. Those downstream pathways include inhibition of nitric oxide synthase (leading to endothelial dysfunction) and activation of vascular endothelial growth factor, plasminogen activator inhibitor-1, transforming growth factor-β, reactive oxygen species, and nuclear factor-κB (the master regulator of inflammation) (Fig. 6.2).[40–42] These toxic pathways downstream of PKC activation, through the induction of vascular dysfunction, growth factors, inflammation, and reactive oxygen species, can be linked to β-cell dysfunction, insulin resistance, and microvascular and macrovascular complications in susceptible individuals with

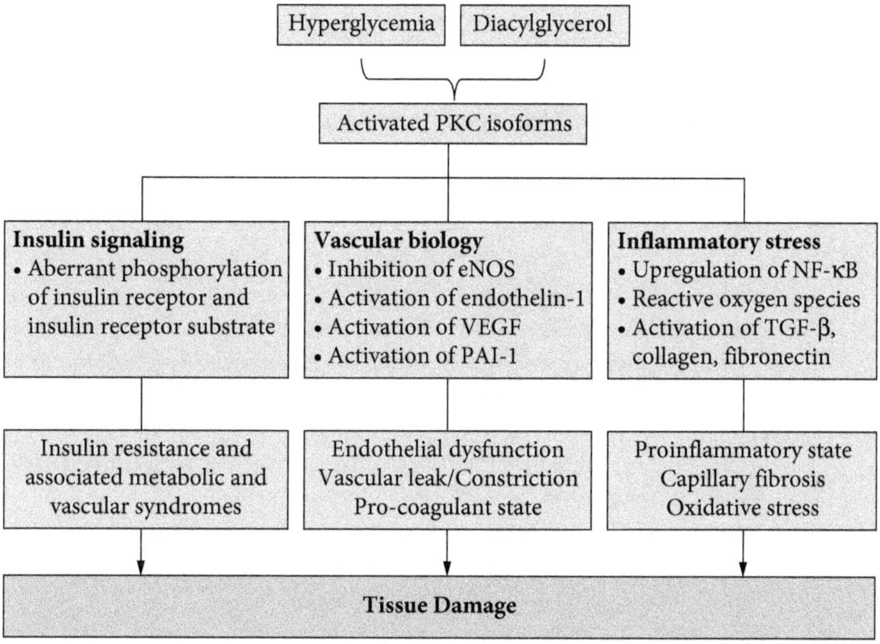

Figure 6.2—Downstream sequelae of hyperglycemia-induced activation of PKC straddle mechanisms that are linked to both microvascular and macrovascular complications.[38,39] eNOS, endothelial nitric oxide synthase; NF-κB, nuclear factor κB; PAI-1, plasminogen activator inhibitor-1; TGF-β, transforming growth factor β; VEGF, vascular endothelial growth factor.

prediabetes.[40] Thus, the current understanding suggests that the modest elevation of blood glucose levels in the prediabetic state may trigger mechanisms that can explain deterioration in glucose tolerance (due to β-cell dysfunction and impaired insulin sensitivity) and progression to type 2 diabetes along with the development of premature vascular complications in susceptible individuals.

References

1. Centers for Disease Control and Prevention. *National Diabetes Statistics Report, 2020. Estimates of Diabetes and Its Burden in the United States.* Atlanta, GA, Centers for Disease Control and Prevention, U.S. Department of Health and Human Services. Available from https://www.cdc.gov/diabetes/pdfs/data/statistics/national-diabetes-statistics-report.pdf. Accessed 28 October 2020

2. Edelstein SL, Knowler WC, Bain, RP, et al. Predictors of progression from impaired glucose tolerance to NIDDM: an analysis of six prospective studies. *Diabetes* 1997;46:701–710
3. Forouhi NG, Luan J, Hennings S, Wareham NJ. Incidence of type 2 diabetes in England and its association with baseline impaired fasting glucose: the Ely study 1990–2000. *Diabet Med* 2007;24:200–207
4. Weyer C, Bogardus C, Mott DM, Pratley RE. The natural history of insulin secretory dysfunction and insulin resistance in the pathogenesis of type 2 diabetes mellitus. *J Clin Invest* 1999;104:787–794
5. Brancati FL, Kao WH, Folsom AR, et al. Incident type 2 diabetes mellitus in African American and white adults: the Atherosclerosis Risk in Communities Study. *JAMA* 2000;283:2253–2259
6. Perseghin G, Ghosh S, Gerow K, Shulman GI. Metabolic defects in lean nondiabetic offspring of NIDDM parents: a cross-sectional study. *Diabetes* 1997;46:1001–1009
7. Gulli G, Ferrannini E, Stern M, et al. The metabolic profile of NIDDM is fully established in glucose-tolerant offspring of two Mexican-American NIDDM parents. *Diabetes* 1992;41:1575–1586
8. Martin BC, Warram JH, Krolewski AS, et al. Role of glucose and insulin resistance in the development of type 2 diabetes mellitus: results of a 25-year follow-up study. *Lancet* 1992;340:925–929
9. Kitabchi AE, Temprosa M, Knowler WC, et al.; Diabetes Prevention Program Research Group. Role of insulin secretion and sensitivity in the evolution of type 2 diabetes in the Diabetes Prevention Program: effects of lifestyle intervention and metformin. *Diabetes* 2005;54:2404–2414
10. Vaag A, Henriksen JE, Madsbad S, et al. Insulin secretion, insulin action and hepatic glucose production in identical twins for non-insulin-dependent diabetes mellitus. *J Clin Invest* 1995;95:690–698
11. Gong Q, Zhang P, Wang J, et al.; Da Qing Diabetes Prevention Study Group. Morbidity and mortality after lifestyle intervention for people with impaired glucose tolerance: 30-year results of the Da Qing Diabetes Prevention Outcome Study. *Lancet Diabetes Endocrinol* 2019;7:452–461
12. Diabetes Prevention Program Research Group. Long-term effects of lifestyle intervention or metformin on diabetes development and microvascular complications over 15-year follow-up: the Diabetes Prevention Program Outcomes Study. *Lancet Diabetes Endocrinol* 2015;3:866–875
13. Tabák AG, Herder C, Rathmann W, et al. Prediabetes: a high-risk state for diabetes development. *Lancet* 2012;379:2279–2290
14. Brannick B, Wynn A, Dagogo-Jack S. Prediabetes as a toxic environment for the initiation of microvascular and macrovascular complications. *Exp Biol Med (Maywood)* 2016;241:1323–1331

15. Piller C. Dubious diagnosis. *Science* 2019;363:1026–1031
16. Lamparter J, Raum P, Pfeiffer N, et al. Prevalence and associations of diabetic retinopathy in a large cohort of prediabetic subjects: the Gutenberg Health Study. *J Diabetes Complications* 2014;28:482–487
17. Papanas N, Vinik AI, Ziegler D. Neuropathy in prediabetes: does the clock start ticking early? *Nat Rev Endocrinol* 2011;7:682–690
18. Ylitalo K, Herman W, Harlow S. Monofilament insensitivity and small and large nerve fiber symptoms in impaired fasting glucose. *Prim Care Diabetes* 2013;7:309–313
19. Diabetes Prevention Program Research Group. The prevalence of retinopathy in impaired glucose tolerance and recent-onset diabetes in the Diabetes Prevention Program. *Diabet Med* 2007;24:137–144
20. Bahar A, Makhlough A, Yousefi A, et al. Correlation between prediabetes conditions and microalbuminuria. *Nephrourol Mon* 2013;5:741–744
21. Plantinga LC, Crews DC, Coresh J, et al.; Centers for Disease Control and Prevention CKD Surveillance Team. Prevalence of chronic kidney disease in US adults with undiagnosed diabetes or prediabetes. *Clin J Am Soc Nephrol* 2010;5:673–682
22. Nguyen TT, Wang JJ, Wong TY. Retinal vascular changes in pre-diabetes and prehypertension: new findings and their research and clinical implications. *Diabetes Care* 2007;30:2708–2715
23. Lott M, Slocomb J, Shivkumar V, et al. Impaired retinal vasodilator responses in prediabetes and type 2 diabetes. *Acta Ophthalmol* 2013;91: e462–e469
24. Eschwege E, Richard JL, Thibult N, et al. Coronary heart disease mortality in relation with diabetes, blood glucose and plasma insulin levels: the Paris Prospective Study, ten years later. *Horm Metab Res Suppl* 1985;15: 41–46
25. Balkau B, Eschwège E, Papoz L, et al. Risk factors for early death in non-insulin dependent diabetes in men with known glucose tolerance status. *BMJ* 1993;307:295–299
26. Ford ES, Zhao G, Li C. Pre-diabetes and the risk for cardiovascular disease: a systematic review of the evidence. *J Am Coll Cardiol* 2010;55: 1310–1317
27. Selvin E, Lazo M, Chen Y, et al. Diabetes mellitus, prediabetes, and incidence of subclinical myocardial damage. *Circulation* 2014;130: 1374–1382
28. Khaw KT, Wareham N, Bingham S, et al. Association of hemoglobin A1c with cardiovascular disease and mortality in adults: the European Prospective Investigation into Cancer in Norfolk. *Ann Intern Med* 2004;14: 413–420

29. Brannick B, Dagogo-Jack S. Prediabetes and cardiovascular disease: pathophysiology and interventions for prevention and risk reduction. *Endocrinol Metab Clin North Am* 2018;47:33–50
30. Stacey RB, Leaverton PE, Schocken DD, et al. Prediabetes and the association with unrecognized myocardial infarction in the Multi-Ethnic Study of Atherosclerosis. *Am Heart J* 2015;170:923–928
31. Roquer J, Rodríguez-Campello A, Cuadrado-Godia E, et al. Ischemic stroke in prediabetic patients. *J Neurol* 2014;261:1866–1870
32. Urabe T, Watada H, Okuma Y, et al. Prevalence of abnormal glucose metabolism and insulin resistance among subtypes of ischemic stroke in Japanese patients. *Stroke* 2009;40:1289–1295
33. Matz K, Keresztes K, Tatschl C, et al. Disorders of glucose metabolism in acute stroke patients: an underrecognized problem. *Diabetes Care* 2006;29:792–797
34. Tanaka R, Ueno Y, Miyamoto N, et al. Impact of diabetes and prediabetes on the short-term prognosis in patients with acute ischemic stroke. *J Neurol Sci* 2013;332:45–50
35. Papa G, Degano C, Iurato MP, et al. Macrovascular complication phenotypes in type 2 diabetic patients. *Cardiovasc Diabetol* 2013;12:20
36. Wang J, Liu L, Zhou Y, et al. Increased fasting glucose and the prevalence of arterial stiffness: a cross-sectional study in Chinese adults. *Neurol Res* 2014;5:427–433
37. Bamberg F, Hetterich H, Rospleszcz S, et al. Subclinical disease burden as assessed by whole-body MRI in subjects with prediabetes, subjects with diabetes, and normal control subjects from the general population: the KORA-MRI Study. *Diabetes* 2017;1:158–169
38. Holman RR, Coleman RL, Chan JCN, et al.; IRIS Trial Investigators. Pioglitazone after ischemic stroke or transient ischemic attack. *N Engl J Med* 2016;374:1321–1331
39. Inzucchi SE, Viscoli CM, Young LH, et al.; IRIS Trial Investigators. Pioglitazone prevents diabetes in insulin-resistant patients with cerebrovascular disease. *Diabetes Care* 2016;39:1684–1692
40. Brownlee M. Banting Lecture 2004: The pathobiology of diabetic complications: a unifying mechanism. *Diabetes* 2005;54:1615–1625
41. Dagogo-Jack S. Chapter 3-Complications of Diabetes Mellitus, in Section 9, Metabolism. In: ACP Medicine, A Publication of the American College of Physicians, Nabel EG (Editor-in-Chief), B C Decker, Inc., Philadelphia, 2010.
42. Dagogo-Jack S. Glycemic control and chronic diabetes complications. In *Therapy for Diabetes Mellitus and Related Disorders*. 6th ed. Umpierrez GE, Ed. Alexandria, VA, American Diabetes Association, 2014, pp. 668–695

Chapter 7

Approach to Prevent Progression from Prediabetes to Type 2 Diabetes

Lifestyle Modification

Some randomized clinical trials, now considered landmark studies, have demonstrated the safety and efficacy of lifestyle modification in preventing or delaying the development of type 2 diabetes in people with prediabetes.[1–5] These landmark studies have the following features in common: *1*) population-based screening to identify individuals with prediabetes; *2*) random assignment of participants to a control group who received standard care or a lifestyle intervention group who attended face-to-face counseling sessions to promote healthy dietary and physical activity habits; and *3*) determination of diabetes incidence in the control and intervention groups and calculation of risk reduction in the latter over a study period ranging from approximately 3 to 6 years. The lifestyle intervention focused on specific goals for diet modification, exercise prescriptions, and weight loss in overweight or obese participants. Specific dietary strategies included calorie reduction (by ~500–1,000 kcal/day), reduction in fat intake limitation (to no more than 30% of total calories), and increased fiber intake. The exercise goal ranged from moderate-intensity physical activity (e.g., brisk walking) for an aggregate of 150 min/week to at least 30 min/day, using aerobic and endurance activities. The weight goals varied from a weight loss of 5–7% of initial body weight or a BMI decrease to <23 kg/m^2. Despite the geographical spread of these studies (North America, Scandinavia, China, and India), all of them showed significant reductions in the incidence of type 2 diabetes when lifestyle intervention was compared with that in control subjects.[1–5] On completion of the active intervention phase, participants in some of the studies were enrolled in long-term follow-up observational studies for the documentation of incident type 2 diabetes and related complications.[6–9] During the extended follow-up phase, body weight tended to converge between the prior lifestyle intervention and control groups, largely because of the weight regain by the former after cessation of active intervention.

Table 7.1—Randomized Controlled Trials of Lifestyle Intervention for Prevention of Type 2 Diabetes in People With Prediabetes[2–5]

Study	Intervention	Number	Mean Age (years)	Mean BMI (kg/m²)	Diabetes Risk Reduction
Da Qing	Diet and exercise	577	46	26	31–46% after 6 years
Finnish DPS	Diet and exercise	522	55	31	58% after 3.2 years
DPP	Diet and exercise or metformin	3,234	54	34	Metformin 31%, lifestyle 58% after 2.8 years
IDDP-1	Lifestyle change plus placebo, or lifestyle change plus metformin	531	46	25.8	Diet and exercise: 28.5%; metformin: 26.4%; diet, exercise, and metformin: 28.2%, after 30 months

DPP, Diabetes Prevention Program; DPS, Diabetes Prevention Study; IDPP-1, Indian Diabetes Prevention Program-1.

Despite the convergence in weight, the long-term data showed a lower cumulative incidence of type 2 diabetes in prior lifestyle intervention recipients compared with the control group.[6–9] The weight regain among the erstwhile lifestyle intervention participants indicates that not all of them were fully habituated to the elements of lifestyle modification. Thus, the continuing diabetes risk reduction reported during long-term follow-up might be indicative of a legacy or the enduring effect of prior lifestyle practices.

The landmark clinical trials that have established lifestyle modification as a safe and effective intervention for preventing progression from prediabetes to type 2 diabetes are summarized in the sections that follow (Table 7.1).

Diabetes Prevention Program

The Diabetes Prevention Program enrolled a multi-ethnic population of 3,234 subjects 25 years or older (mean age 51 years) from 27 centers in the United States Enrollment criteria included high-normal or impaired fasting plasma glucose (95–125 mg/dL) and documentation of impaired glucose tolerance (2-h plasma glucose >140 to <200 mg/dL) along with BMI >25 kg/m² (>22 kg/m² for Asian Americans). Participants were randomly assigned to placebo, metformin, or a lifestyle intervention program.[3] Individuals assigned to the intensive lifestyle intervention group were provided an individualized, flexible, and culturally sensitive

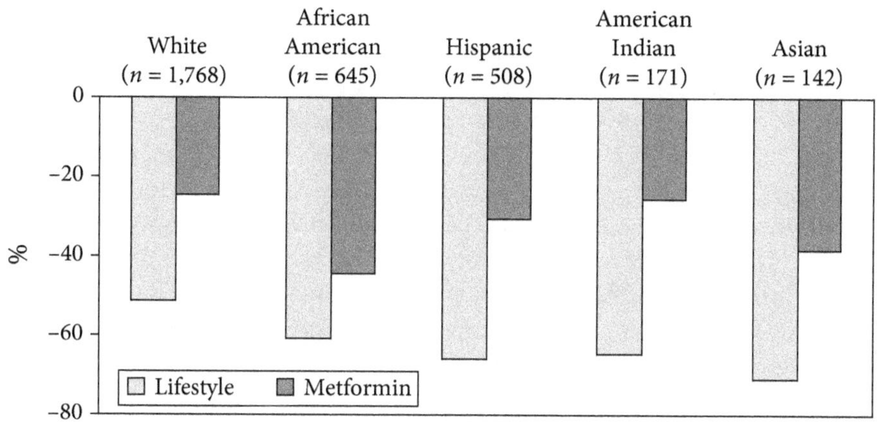

Figure 7.1—Diabetes risk reduction in active intervention arms relative to placebo among participants in the Diabetes Prevention Program from different ethnic groups.[3]

16-lesson curriculum, administered by case managers and designed to help these participants achieve the following goals: at least 7% weight reduction, consumption of a low-calorie/low-fat diet, and at least 150 min/week of moderate physical activity (similar in intensity to brisk walking).

After an average follow-up period of 2.8 years, the incidence of diabetes was 11.0 and 4.8 cases per 100 person-years in the placebo and lifestyle groups, respectively, yielding risk reduction of 58% in the intensive lifestyle intervention group relative to control subjects. The metformin treatment group showed a 31% reduction in type 2 diabetes incidence when compared with the control group.[3] The lifestyle intervention was well tolerated, and beneficial effects were observed in all subgroups (older vs. younger, obese vs. nonobese, and all ethnic groups). Figure 7.1 shows the relative reduction in diabetes incidence in the metformin and lifestyle groups among Diabetes Prevention Program participants from different ethnic groups. Long-term follow-up of the Diabetes Prevention Program cohort has shown continued diabetes risk reduction in the active treatment arms: during a mean follow-up of 15 years, the incidence of type 2 diabetes decreased by 27% in the lifestyle intervention group and by 18% in the metformin group, compared with the placebo group.[8] This durability of the protective effect of lifestyle modification, >10 years after cessation of active intervention, has been referred to as a "legacy" effect.

Da Qing study

The Da Qing study screened 110,660 men and women from 33 health care clinics in the city of Da Qing, China, and enrolled 577 subjects with impaired glucose tolerance.[2] Using cluster randomization, the clinics were assigned to provide participants with one of three interventions (dietary modification only, exercise only, or diet plus exercise) or to serve as a control for 6 years. At baseline, the participants had a mean age of 45 years and a mean BMI of 26 kg/m^2.

The dietary advice was tailored to baseline BMI classification, with a target BMI of <23 kg/m^2; the exercise goal was to increase physical activity by 1–2 units per day, defined by time and intensity of exercise. Individual and group counseling sessions were held approximately every 2 weeks during the first 3 months and quarterly thereafter for the remainder of the study. The primary end point (cumulative incidence of type 2 diabetes at 6 years) occurred in 67.7% of subjects in the control group, 43.8% in the diet-only group, 41.1% in the exercise-only group, and 46% in the diet-plus-exercise group. Because of the use of BMI stratification for the dietary intervention, outcomes data were examined by enrollment BMI: the incidence rate of type 2 diabetes in participants with baseline BMI <25 kg/m^2 was similar to the rate seen in participants with BMI ≥25 kg/m^2.[2] Thus, the efficacy of lifestyle intervention was seen in lean as well as overweight subjects. Compared with control, the adjusted diabetes risk reduction for the diet, exercise, and diet-plus-exercise intervention groups were 31, 46, and 42% respectively.[2] Notably, the diet-plus-exercise group did not show additive benefit when compared to the diet-only and exercise-only groups. In subsequent analyses, all lifestyle groups were combined and compared with the control group.[2]

Active intervention ceased after 6 years, but the cohort continues to be followed up. The Da Qing investigators reported outcomes ascertained in 2006 (20 years), 2009 (23 years), and, most recently, 2016 (30 years). During each of these extended follow-up time points, diabetes incidence remained significantly lower in the lifestyle intervention groups compared with the control group.[7,9–12]

Finnish Diabetes Prevention Study

The Finnish Diabetes Prevention Study enrolled 522 middle-aged, overweight subjects (mean age 55 years, mean BMI 31 kg/m^2) with documented impaired glucose tolerance.[4] The participants were randomized to either a usual care control group or to an intensive lifestyle intervention group. The intensive lifestyle intervention group attended seven individual nutritional and exercise counseling sessions during the first year, followed by quarterly sessions for the remainder of the study. The goals of lifestyle intervention included weight loss of ≥5% (not to exceed 0.5–1 kg/week) through reduction in the consumption of total fat and saturated fat along with increased fiber intake and increased physical activity by ~210 min/week. As reported by the investigators, the lifestyle intervention group reported less sedentary behavior, decreased fat intake, and increased consumption of dietary fiber intake than the control group at 1 and 3 years, and they also lost more weight

(~4 vs. ~1 kg). The cumulative incidence of type 2 diabetes after 4 years was 11% in the lifestyle intervention group and 23% in the control group. The diabetes risk reduction was 58% in the lifestyle intervention group compared to the control group during the active phase of the study; the risk reduction was 39% 9 years after cessation of lifestyle intervention.[4,6]

Indian Diabetes Prevention Program

The Indian Diabetes Prevention Program-1, conducted in Chennai, India, randomized subjects with impaired glucose tolerance to a control group (with standard advice) ($N = 136$), lifestyle modification group ($N = 133$), metformin treatment group ($N = 133$), and lifestyle modification plus metformin treatment group ($N = 136$).[5] The mean age of the participants was 45.9 ± 5.7 years, and their mean BMI was 25.8 ± 3.5 kg/m^2. The lifestyle modification intervention used counseling sessions aimed at promoting healthy eating habits (decreased consumption of refined carbohydrates and fats and increased intake of dietary fiber) and a physical activity goal of at least 30 minutes daily. After a median follow-up of 30 months, the incidence of diabetes was reduced by 28.5% in the lifestyle group, 26.4% in the metformin group, and 28.2% in the lifestyle modification plus metformin group, compared with the control group.[5] These results were observed despite the lack of significant weight change in the two groups that focused on lifestyle change. The effect of metformin was not additive to that of lifestyle modification.[5]

Effect of Lifestyle Intervention on Microvascular and Macrovascular Complications

Given the efficacy of lifestyle intervention in preventing or delaying the development of type 2 diabetes, it seems intuitive to expect that a corresponding protection against the development of complications, especially microvascular complications, are closely linked to hyperglycemia. However, data from 10 years of follow-up of participants in the Finnish Diabetes Prevention Study did not find a decrease in cardiovascular disease mortality in the prior lifestyle intervention group (compared to usual care), despite evidence of continued reduction in type 2 diabetes incidence in the lifestyle group.[13] Similarly, prior lifestyle intervention was not associated with a uniform reduction in the incidence of microvascular complications after 15 years of follow-up of the overall Diabetes Prevention Program cohort.[8] (Women, but not men, in the Diabetes Prevention Program lifestyle group experienced a significant reduction in microvascular complications after 15 years.) The Diabetes Prevention Program investigators[21] assessed the effects of lifestyle intervention, metformin, and placebo on cardiovascular disease risk factors and markers of the metabolic syndrome among the subjects with impaired glucose tolerance enrolled in the study.[14–16] Compared with the placebo and metformin arms, subjects assigned to lifestyle intervention showed decreased blood pressure, increased HDL cholesterol levels, and lower triglyceride levels during approximately 3 years of follow-up. Intensive lifestyle modification also was associated with a reduction in the more atherogenic small, dense LDL particles and overall manifestations of the metabolic syndrome.[14,15]

Furthermore, there was a reduction in the use of medications for treating hypertension or dyslipidemia among lifestyle subjects compared with the other groups. Besides reducing the need for antihypertensive medications, lifestyle intervention was associated with a marked reduction in new cases of hypertension in the Diabetes Prevention Program. The prevalence of hypertension at baseline was ~30% in the three comparison groups. After 3 years of follow-up, the prevalence increased to ~40% in the placebo and metformin arms but remained at ~30% in the intensive lifestyle group, which represents a risk reduction of 33% in the lifestyle group, compared with placebo or metformin treatment.[14,15] This finding is in agreement with the well-known favorable effect of exercise, dietary modification, and weight loss on the regulation of blood pressure.

The 20-year follow-up report from the Da Qing study showed a significant decrease in the incidence of severe retinopathy (but not nephropathy, neuropathy, or cardiovascular disease) among lifestyle participants compared to control subjects.[9] However, on further follow-up of the Da Qing cohort for 23 years, the investigators reported that participants in the prior lifestyle intervention group showed a significant reduction, not only in the cumulative diabetes incidence, but also in the occurrence of cardiovascular disease death and all-cause mortality, compared with the control group.[10] Those results were strengthened by the 30-year follow-up data from the Da Qing cohort.[11] Compared with the control group, prior lifestyle intervention was associated with reductions in the cumulative incidence of diabetes, microvascular complications, cardiovascular disease events, and cardiovascular disease as well as all-cause mortality.[11] The effect size of the risk reductions with lifestyle ranged from 26 to 35% across the various outcomes. With such magnitudes of risk reduction, the number needed to prevent one death during 30 years of follow-up was only 10 people with impaired glucose tolerance.

It is rare for medical interventions to have such a remarkable longevity benefit. For comparison, ~250 people would need to be treated with a statin drug for 1–6 years to prevent one death in a high-risk primary prevention cohort.[17] Based on the 30-year results from the Da Qing study, longer-term follow-up of other diabetes prevention cohorts[8] and the Finnish Diabetes Prevention Study[13] may be required to demonstrate more robust data regarding prevention of microvascular complications.

The extraordinary cardiovascular and mortality benefits of lifestyle intervention observed after 30 years of follow-up of the Da Qing cohort are intriguing.

Although the Da Qing investigators suggested that the effect of lifestyle intervention in delaying the onset of diabetes could explain the difference in clinical outcomes observed in the control and intervention groups, the median delay in diabetes onset in the lifestyle intervention group was 3.96 years.[11] It is unlikely that a 4-year delay in the onset of type 2 diabetes can result in the 26–35% reductions in the risks of microvascular and macrovascular complications and cardiovascular and all-cause mortality. Randomized, controlled studies that enrolled subjects with recent-onset or long-standing type 2 diabetes have not reported such cardiovascular disease or mortality benefits from aggressive glycemic control.[18]

Thus, other nonglycemic factors resulting from or associated with the lifestyle modification could have contributed to the benefits observed in the lifestyle arm of the Da Qing study.[11] One such factor is smoking: at baseline, Da Qing participants in the lifestyle intervention group reported higher smoking rates than participants in the control group (50 vs. 39%).[11] A possible spillover impact of frequent lifestyle counseling sessions on smoking habit is conceivable, and smoking cessation could decrease microvascular and macrovascular risks.[19–21] Blood pressure control is another nonglycemic mediator of the vascular benefits observed in the lifestyle arm of the Da Qing study. (After 30 years of follow-up, systolic blood pressure was 4.2 mmHg lower and diastolic blood pressure was 3.2 mmHg lower in the lifestyle intervention group compared with the control group.[11]) For reference, decreases of 10 mmHg in systolic blood pressure and 5 mmHg in diastolic blood pressure were associated with decreases of 32% in diabetes-related deaths, 44% in strokes, and 37% in microvascular complications in the UK Prospective Diabetes Study.[22] The Da Qing study cohort was not overweight, so weight loss may not have been a major protective mechanism; however, lifestyle modification could decrease visceral fat and thereby improve cardiometabolic health. Finally, even without weight loss, increased physical activity improves cardiorespiratory fitness, a significant predictor of cardiovascular health and longevity.[23,24] Notably, improved cardiorespiratory fitness from moderate-intensity physical activity training could have lasting benefits 10 years after cessation of the intervention.[24] Thus, historical lifestyle intervention among the subjects with prediabetes enrolled in the Da Qing study appeared to have had profound legacy effects that were evident 30 years later (i.e., 24 years after cessation of active intervention).

Children and Adolescents

A major limitation of these studies is the exclusion of individuals younger than age 25 years. The surging prevalence of type 2 diabetes in children and adolescents requires that the efficacy of diabetes prevention strategies be demonstrated in younger age-groups.[25–30] Obesity and physical inactivity are major risk factors for type 2 diabetes in children (as in adults); additional risk factors in young individuals include female sex, ethnicity, family history of type 2 diabetes, peripubertal age, and intrauterine exposure to diabetes.[25–30] Unchecked, the increasing rates of type 2 diabetes in children and adolescents predict dire consequences (especially microvascular complications and cardiovascular disease) for these young people at the prime of their youth. Primary prevention of childhood type 2 diabetes, therefore, is of utmost public health importance. Programs aimed at screening and recognition of children and adolescents with prediabetes would facilitate the targeting of preventive interventions.

In 2003, the National Institute of Diabetes and Digestive and Kidney Diseases (NIDDK) launched an initiative to fund a multicenter school-based trial to prevent the development of type 2 diabetes in children in middle school.[31] That program identified widespread obesity and decreased physical activity as the likely key susceptibility factors for type 2 diabetes in youth and rightly focused on a behavioral approach. It was noted that children in the sixth to eighth grade (middle school) are generally 11–14 years old, and most are going through puberty, a time when the risk of obesity is markedly increased. The adolescent period also is noted as a time when children tend to increasingly take greater responsibility for their food choices, eating patterns, and exercise habits.[31] Thus, a school-based intervention aimed at modifying dietary and physical activity practices of adolescents could potentially decrease sedentariness, increase physical activity, optimize food habits, and help reduce the risk of overweight/obesity. The successful prevention or reversal of obesity in youth would have the metabolic effects of decreasing obesity-related insulin resistance, which should improve glucose tolerance and decrease the risks of prediabetes and diabetes.

The NIDDK-sponsored study, HEALTHY, evaluated the effects of a 3-year, multicomponent, school-based program on risk factors for type 2 diabetes in 4,603 children (52.7% girls) who were followed from sixth grade through eighth grade.[32] Using a cluster design, 42 schools were randomly assigned to either a multicomponent school-based intervention (21 schools) or a control group, comprising assessment only (21 schools). Students enrolled in sixth grade were eligible for participation if they did not have diabetes or limitations to engage in physical activity. The mean (± SD) age of the students at enrollment was 11.3 ± 0.6 years, and their ethnic composition was 54.2% Hispanic, 19.3% white, 18.0% black, and 8.5% "other." At baseline, ~50% of the students had BMI ≥85th percentile and ~30% had BMI ≥95th percentile, and their fasting glucose level was 93.5 mg/dL.[32]

The integrated lifestyle modification intervention focused on healthy eating patterns, increasing moderate-to-vigorous physical activity, behavioral skills (including self-monitoring and goal-setting), and communication strategies and social marketing.[32] Social marketing is a carefully designed strategy, based on commercial marketing principles and techniques, that aims to induce and maintain long-term change in human behavior. The primary outcome was the combined overweight and obesity prevalence (BMI ≥85th percentile); prespecified secondary outcomes were obesity (BMI ≥95th percentile), BMI *z* score, waist circumference, and fasting glucose and insulin levels. The baseline measurements were performed on location at the schools in the fall of 2006 (sixth grade), and follow-up measurements occurred in the spring of 2009 (eighth grade). The results showed a decrease in the primary outcome (prevalence of overweight plus obesity) among students in the intervention and control schools, without a significant difference between them.[32] However, the secondary outcomes favored intervention: the reductions in BMI *z* score, percentage of students with waist circumference at or above the 90th percentile, fasting insulin levels, and obesity prevalence were all greater in the intervention schools versus measurement-only (control) schools.[32] Notably, the decrease in the prevalence of obesity in the intervention schools was particularly pronounced in the subgroup of students with excess body weight at the time of joining the study. There was no significant change in fasting glucose among students in intervention or control schools; the mean fasting glucose remained in the tight range of 93–94 mg/dL throughout the study.[32]

Interestingly, even among the 49.3% of children in the control schools who were overweight or obese at baseline, the prevalence of combined overweight and obesity deceased by 15.9%, and that of obesity deceased by 8.5% at the end of the study.[32] Those impressive results were probably due, at least in part, to the Hawthorne effect of participation in the study and undergoing assessments.[33–35] Also, the feedback on each measurement given to parents of children in the study could have triggered changes in domestic dietary and lifestyle decisions.

The HEALTHY study demonstrated the feasibility of a school-based intervention program to improve health behavior among adolescents. The results were generally positive and encouraging, despite the nontargeted approach in the inclusion of participants. Arguably, focusing on the segment with higher risk factors (such as obesity, family history of diabetes, and habitual physical inactivity) would have produced even more impressive results. Nonetheless, significant reduction in adiposity and insulin resistance (as indicated by lower fasting insulinemia) observed in the intervention group should decrease the risks of dysglycemia, prediabetes, and type 2 diabetes.

Mechanisms and Mediators of Diabetes Prevention by Lifestyle Intervention

To explore explanatory mechanisms for the efficacy of lifestyle intervention, the Finnish Diabetes Prevention Study investigators compared insulin sensitivity and insulin secretion at baseline ($N = 87$) and after 4 years ($N = 52$) in subjects from a matched group of participants in the lifestyle intervention and control arms of the study cohort.[36] After 4 years of follow-up, weight and waist circumference decreases were greater in the intervention group than in the control group. A strong correlation was observed between the 4-year changes in insulin sensitivity and weight: insulin sensitivity improved by 64% in the highest tertile of weight loss, whereas a 24% deterioration was observed in the lowest tertile. Acute insulin secretory response to glucose during a frequently sampled intravenous glucose tolerance test declined significantly in the control group but was preserved in the lifestyle intervention group.[36]

In a similar analysis, insulin sensitivity and insulin secretion were assessed at baseline and 1 year post-intervention among Diabetes Prevention Program participants assigned to the placebo group (N = 1,082), lifestyle intervention group (N = 1,079), and metformin treatment group (N = 1,073).[37] The findings showed that progression from prediabetes to type 2 diabetes was inversely associated with baseline insulin sensitivity and baseline insulin secretion. Post-intervention, the improvement in insulin sensitivity was associated with decreased hazard of progression from prediabetes to type 2 diabetes in all treatment arms (hazard rate ratio 0.29–0.79 per SD increase).[37] The improvement in insulin secretion was also associated with decreased risk of type 2 diabetes in all treatment arms (hazard rate ratio 0.46–0.95 per SD increase).[37] Compared with the metformin and placebo groups, individuals assigned to the intensive lifestyle intervention arm showed the greatest 1-year post-intervention improvement in insulin sensitivity and the best preservation of β-cell function.[37] No significant temporal changes in insulin sensitivity and β-cell function were seen in the control group. The changes in insulin sensitivity and insulin secretion observed in the metformin treatment group were intermediate between individuals in the lifestyle intervention and placebo groups. Circulating proinsulin level (a marker of β-cell stress) also strongly predicted diabetes, with lower proinsulin predicting a lower hazard of type 2 diabetes in all Diabetes Prevention Program treatment arms.[37]

In the Diabetes Prevention Program, weight loss was significantly associated with decreased incidence of type 2 diabetes, and baseline weight was inversely correlated with insulin sensitivity ($r = -0.4$) and insulin secretion ($r = -0.4$) after adjustment for age, sex, and race/ethnicity.[37] Assessment 1 year post-intervention showed that the change in insulin sensitivity was also inversely associated with weight ($r = 0.33$) after adjustment for age, sex, and race/ethnicity.[37] In multivariate models that included changes in weight, insulin sensitivity, and insulin secretion, each variable significantly and independently predicted progression to type 2 diabetes, after adjusting for the other two variables.[37] These findings demonstrate that the robust reduction in diabetes incidence achieved in the Diabetes Prevention Program lifestyle intervention group can be explained by their higher baseline values and post-intervention improvements in insulin secretion and sensitivity along with greater weight loss relative to the placebo and metformin treatment groups.[37] In a further analysis, the Diabetes Prevention Program investigators explored the contribution of changes in weight, diet, and physical activity on the risk of progression from prediabetes to type 2 diabetes among the participants assigned to intensive lifestyle intervention (N = 1,079; mean age 50.6 years, BMI 33.9 kg/m^2), using Cox proportional hazards regression over 3.2 years of follow-up.[38] The findings showed that weight loss was the dominant predictor of decreased type 2 diabetes hazard among intensive lifestyle participants. The hazard ratio associated with each per 5-kg weight loss was 0.42 (95% CI 0.35–0.51, $P < 0.0001$). After adjusting for changes in diet and physical activity, each 1-kg weight loss predicted a 16% reduction in diabetes risk.[38] Congruently, the magnitude of weight loss was positively correlated with decreased consumption of fat and increased physical activity.[38] Furthermore, increased physical activity was an important mechanism for sustaining weight loss and preventing regain.[38] Notably, among 495 participants who did not meet the weight loss target at year 1, the subgroup who achieved the physical activity target of ≥150 min/week experienced a 44% decrease on diabetes incidence.[38]

Additional mechanisms/mediators of the beneficial effects of lifestyle intervention on diabetes risk include decreased proinflammatory cytokines,[39] upregulation of adiponectin,[40] and improvements in blood pressure and lipid profile[14,15,41] (Fig. 7.2). In the Diabetes Prevention Program, the lifestyle intervention group who showed the greatest risk reduction for progression to type 2 diabetes also had significant decreases in proinflammatory markers[39] and significantly higher adiponectin levels.[40] Among the Diabetes Prevention Program participants, each 3-μg/mL increase in adiponectin level predicted a 39% lower diabetes hazard in the lifestyle group, a 24% lower hazard in the metformin group, and a 21% lower hazard in the placebo group. During follow-up, the highest increase in adiponectin occurred in the lifestyle intervention arm (0.83 ± 0.05 μg/mL) compared with 0.23 ± 0.05 μg/mL in the metformin arm and 0.10 ± 0.05 μg/mL in the placebo group.[40] The increases in adiponectin were independently associated with reduction in progression from prediabetes to type 2 diabetes in the lifestyle group. In the Cox proportional hazards models, each ~1 μg/mL increase in adiponectin was associated with a 16% (95% CI 1.0–28) reduction in the rate of progression to type 2 diabetes in participants randomized to receive the lifestyle intervention, after adjusting for age, sex, race, baseline weight, baseline adiponectin, and change in weight.[40]

Other emerging or putative contributory mechanisms include plausible impacts of lifestyle modification and weight loss on the metabolome, microbiome, microRNAs, and gene expression.[42–44]

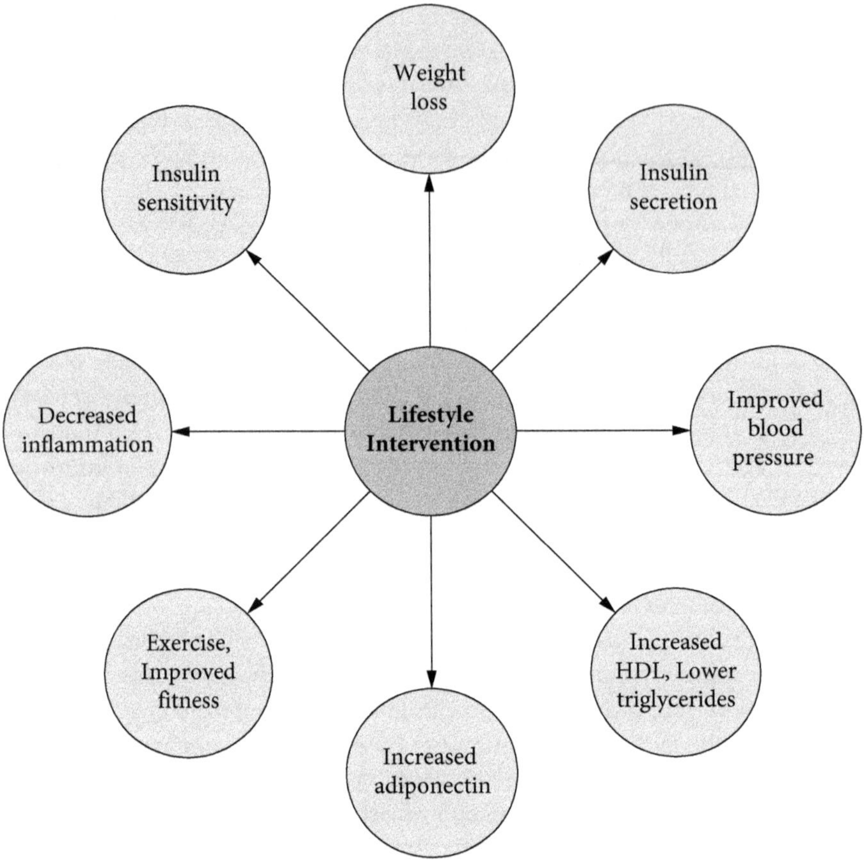

Figure 7.2—Mechanisms and mediators of diabetes prevention with lifestyle modification.

Diabetes Risk-Conferring Genes and Lifestyle Intervention

Data from the Diabetes Prevention Program and Finnish Diabetes Prevention Study suggest that lifestyle modification could have attenuated genetic risk for type 2 diabetes. Analysis of polymorphisms in the promoter region of the *TNF*-α gene in the entire cohort showed that participants in the Finnish Diabetes Prevention Study who harbored the –308A allele (G-308A and A-308A genotypes) had a higher incidence of type 2 diabetes compared with individuals harboring the GG genotype.[45] When the lifestyle intervention and control groups were analyzed separately, the presence of the –308A allele of the *TNF*-α gene predicted incident diabetes only in the lifestyle intervention group. Despite showing similar weight loss, the incidence of type 2 diabetes was lower in lifestyle participants with the

GG polymorphism compared with participants harboring the −308A allele (odds ratio 1.80 [95% CI 1.05–3.09], $P = 0.034$).[45] The 3-year incidence of type 2 diabetes among carriers of the −308A allele was 20.8% in the control group and 5% in the lifestyle intervention group.[45]

The Pro12Ala polymorphism of the *PPAR-γ* gene was also examined in relation to weight gain and incident type 2 diabetes in the Finnish cohort.[45] After 3 years of follow-up, participants harboring the Ala12 allele were two-fold more likely to have progressed from prediabetes to type 2 diabetes compared with subjects having the Pro12Pro genotype (odds ratio 2.11 [95% CI 1.20–3.72], $P = 0.010$).[45] However, the increased diabetes risk conferred by the Ala12 allele appeared confined to the control group, and no subjects with the Ala12Ala genotype reportedly progressed to type 2 diabetes.[45] It was noted that lifestyle intervention resulted in significantly greater weight loss in subjects with the Ala12Ala genotype than in individuals with the Pro12Pro genotype. The investigators concluded that the Ala12 allele increases the risk of type 2 diabetes in obese subjects with prediabetes, but lifestyle modification and weight loss markedly attenuate the diabetogenic effect of the Ala12 allele, possibly because of an improved insulin sensitivity. While these results are intriguing, the rather small number of diabetes events (19 subjects in the lifestyle intervention group and 50 subjects in the control group developed type 2 diabetes during the 3-year follow-up) should temper enthusiasm regarding the findings. The Diabetes Prevention Program investigators also observed increased risk of incident type 2 diabetes among participants with the Ala12 polymorphism but found no interaction with interventions.[46] However, it was noted that among Diabetes Prevention Program participants assigned to lifestyle intervention, body fat decreased across genotypes, but the reduction was greater in Ala12 carriers.[46]

In the Diabetes Prevention Program, 3,548 study subjects with prediabetes at baseline were genotyped for *TCF7L2* variants, and the effects of *TCF7L2* alleles on incident type 2 diabetes and measures of insulin secretion and insulin sensitivity (at baseline and at one year) were examined.[47] During a follow-up period of 3 years, participants in the placebo group homozygous for the risk allele in rs7903146 (TT genotype) had an 81% higher hazard of developing type 2 diabetes than participants harboring the CC genotype (hazard ratio 1.81 [95% CI 1.21–2.70], $P = 0.004$). Among participants receiving lifestyle intervention, the diabetes hazard for TT carriers was not significantly different from the hazard among carriers of the CC genotype (hazard ratio 1.15 [95% CI 0.68–1.94], $P = 0.60$), and the corresponding hazard ratio among the metformin treatment group was 1.62 (95% 1.03–2.54; $P = 0.04$) (Fig. 7.3). On further exploration, the TT genotype was associated with decreased insulin secretion but not increased insulin resistance at baseline.[47] Comparable results were obtained for the risk allele in rs12255372 of the *TCF7L2* gene, and the observations were consistent across sex and race/ethnicity.[47] The Diabetes Prevention Program investigators interpreted

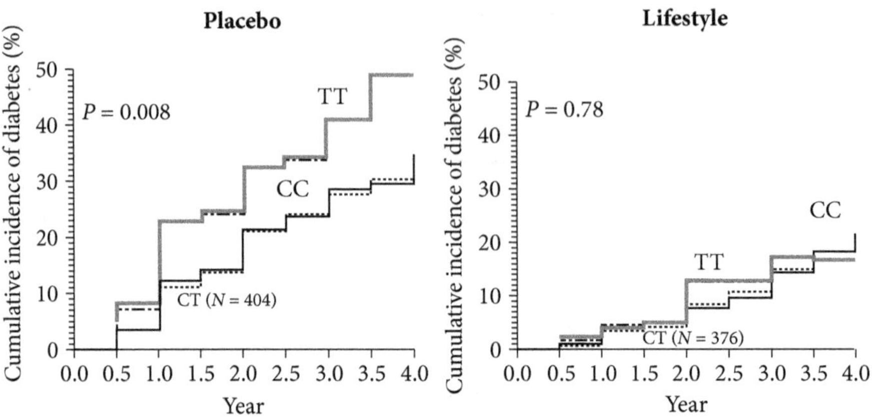

Figure 7.3—*TCF7L2* polymorphisms and progression to diabetes among participants assigned to the placebo and lifestyle intervention groups in the Diabetes Prevention Program. Compared with participants harboring the CC genotype, carriers of the TT genotype had an 81% higher hazard of developing type 2 diabetes if assigned to a placebo but a similar and much lower hazard if assigned to a lifestyle intervention.[48]

the failure to detect a significant diabetogenic effect of the *TCF7L2* genotype in the lifestyle intervention group as possible evidence that a behavioral intervention can mitigate the risk conferred by genetic background. Somewhat similar observations have been made regarding polymorphisms of the ectoenzyme nucleotide pyrophosphatase phosphodiesterase 1 (*ENPP1*) gene and incident type 2 diabetes in the Diabetes Prevention Program cohort.[48] *ENPP1* inhibits insulin signaling, and the Q allele in the K121Q polymorphism confers increased risk for type 2 diabetes.[48] Among Diabetes Prevention Program participants, carriers of the Q allele had a 38% greater risk of progression from prediabetes to type 2 diabetes compared to KK homozygotes. Like the observation regarding the risk allele of *TCF7L2*, the effect of the Q allele of the *ENPP1* gene was markedly attenuated among participants assigned to lifestyle intervention[48] (Table 7.2).

Taken together, these data underscore the rationale for targeting weight loss as a primary strategy for diabetes prevention in overweight or obese individuals with prediabetes. Increased physical activity is an important adjunct for maintaining weight loss; high levels of activity can also contribute to diabetes prevention, despite suboptimal weight loss. Current understanding supports the notion that weight loss, dietary modification, and increased levels of physical activity improve glucoregulation and prevent the progression from prediabetes to diabetes via multiple mechanisms that involve physiological, biochemical, molecular, and possibly genomic and epigenetic pathways that are beneficial for cardiometabolic health.

Table 7.2—Gene by Lifestyle Interactions in Diabetes Prevention Studies

Gene	Metabolic Outcome	Risk Reduction by Lifestyle Intervention vs. Placebo	Source
TCF7L2	Type 2 diabetes	66%	DPP[37]
ENPP1	Type 2 diabetes	53%	DPP[48]
TNF-α (−308A allele vs. G308G genotype)*	Type 2 diabetes	80%	FDPS[45]
PPAR-γ (Pro12Ala genotype)	Obesity	20%	DPP[46]

DPP, Diabetes Prevention Program; FDPS, Finnish Diabetes Prevention Study. *The tumor necrosis factor (TNF)-α polymorphism predicted diabetes in the lifestyle arm only.

Limitations of lifestyle intervention

Lifestyle intervention programs have generally been designed as randomized controlled efficacy trials and conducted predominantly at research centers. These trials have involved frequent in-person visits and deployed sizeable staff, comprising a multidisciplinary team of physicians, nurses, dietitians, psychologists, exercise physiologists, and other support personnel. Substantial resources and support from funding agencies were needed for execution of these studies, and services were offered at no cost to the study subjects, many of whom actually received stipends for their participation. Thus, it is necessary to determine whether the impressive diabetes risk reduction achieved in the randomized controlled trials is translatable in routine clinical practice and community settings. In that regard, many community initiatives have demonstrated the feasibility of community translation of diabetes prevention programs.[49-51] The subject of community translation of diabetes prevention is discussed further in Chapter 9.

Medications for Diabetes Prevention

Intervention studies have reported a relative reduction in the risk of incident diabetes from lifestyle modification that ranges from ~25% to ~60%.[1-5] The substantial number of individuals with residual risk of incident diabetes, despite lifestyle intervention, begs the question as to whether medications have a role for preventing the development of diabetes among people with prediabetes, particularly individuals for whom lifestyle changes have failed to halt glycemic progression. Another pertinent question is whether medications should be considered in individuals with prediabetes who are unable or unwilling to implement the optimal levels of weight loss, dietary changes, and physical activity that have been demonstrated to prevent progression to type 2 diabetes. The U.S. Food and Drug Administration has not approved any drug specifically for the treatment of prediabetes or prevention of progression to diabetes. However, numerous medications have been tested in randomized controlled trials for their efficacy on incident type 2 diabetes in people with prediabetes[3,5,52–61] (Table 7.3). Also, some drugs approved for treatment of obesity have analyzed subgroups for the outcome of incident diabetes and reported substantial benefits.[62,63] In general, the medications that have been tested in randomized controlled trials showed variable efficacy on diabetes prevention (~25–70% risk reduction vs. placebo), were associated with adverse effects that caused many participants to drop out, and were only effective during the period of administration. In the studies that formally assessed the effects of withdrawal of metformin, rosiglitazone, or pioglitazone, a rebound in blood glucose occurred, indicating attenuation of the pharmacological effects of the medications.[59–61]

Investigators in the Study to Prevent Non-Insulin-Dependent Diabetes Mellitus (STOP-NIDDM) randomized subjects with prediabetes to treatment with α-glucosidase inhibitor acarbose (100 mg three times daily) or a placebo and reported a 25% relative reduction in progression to type 2 diabetes in the acarbose group during a mean follow-up period of 3.3 years.[52] Nearly one-quarter of participants dropped out of the study (half of them doing so during the first year), mostly because of gastrointestinal side effects.[52] In the Xenical in the Prevention of Diabetes in Obese Subjects (XENDOS) study, 3,305 obese subjects with normal glucose tolerance (79%) or prediabetes (21%) were randomly assigned to lifestyle modification plus treatment with the pancreatic lipase inhibitor orlistat (120 mg three times daily) or placebo.[53] After 4 years of follow-up, a significantly greater weight loss occurred in the orlistat group than the placebo group (5.8 vs. 3.0 kg), and the cumulative incidence of diabetes was 9.0% with the placebo and 6.2% with orlistat, yielding to a relative risk reduction of 37.3%.[53] Exploratory analyses showed that the diabetes risk reduction was largely explained by posttreatment reclassification of subjects enrolled with prediabetes.[53]

Thiazolidinedione drugs have been evaluated for diabetes prevention in several studies, including the Diabetes Reduction Assessment with Ramipril and Rosiglitazone Medication (DREAM)[54] trial, the Actos Now for the Prevention of Diabetes (ACT NOW) trial,[55] and the Indian Diabetes Prevention Program-2.[56] Further, the Canadian Normoglycemia Outcomes Evaluation (CANOE) trial used a strategy of low-dose metformin in combination with low-dose rosiglitazone.[57] Collectively, these studies showed diabetes risk reduction rates of >50–75% with thiazolidinedione drugs compared with a placebo. Adverse drug effects, including weight gain and heart failure, were reported.[54,55] In the CANOE trial, low doses of metformin (500 mg twice daily) and rosiglitazone (2 mg daily), used in combination, resulted in a 66% decrease in incident type 2 diabetes relative to a placebo

Table 7.3—Randomized Controlled Trials of Medications for Prevention of Type 2 Diabetes in People with Prediabetes[2–5]

Study	Intervention	*n*	Mean Age (years)	Mean BMI (kg/m²)	Diabetes Risk Reduction
STOP-NIDDM	Acarbose	1,429	55	31	25%, after 3.3 years
DPP	Diet and exercise or metformin	3,234	54	34	Metformin 31%, lifestyle 58%, after 2.8 years
Xendos	Orlistat plus diet plus exercise	3,305 (21% with IGT)	43	31	Entire group 37%, IGT subgroup 45%, after 4 years
DREAM	Rosiglitazone	5,269	54.7	30.9	62% after ~3 years
IDPP-1	Lifestyle change plus placebo or lifestyle change plus metformin	531	46	25.8	Diet and exercise: 28.5%; metformin: 26.4%; diet, exercise, and metformin: 28.2%, after 30 months
CANOE	Combination rosiglitazone and metformin vs. placebo	207	50	31.3	26% in the combination group, after 3.9 years
ACT NOW	Pioglitazone	602	53	33	72% with pioglitazone over 2.4 years

ACT NOW, Actos Now for the Prevention of Diabetes; CANOE, Canadian Normoglycemia Outcomes Evaluation; DPP, Diabetes Prevention Program; DREAM, Diabetes Reduction Assessment with Ramipril and Rosiglitazone Medication; IDPP-1, Indian Diabetes Prevention Program-1; STOP-NIDDM, Study to Prevent Non-Insulin-Dependent Diabetes Mellitus.

among subjects enrolled with impaired glucose tolerance. The low doses were reportedly well tolerated, without clinically relevant adverse events.[57] A 5-year trial of nateglinide and valsartan (NAVIGATOR) versus a placebo, using a 2 × 2 factorial design, along with lifestyle modification, showed a modest 14% reduction in incident type 2 diabetes among prediabetes subjects treated with valsartan, but nateglinide was not better than a placebo.[58]

The inclusion of the medication arm along with lifestyle intervention and placebo treatment in some diabetes prevention trials enables direct comparison between the effects of medication versus those of lifestyle intervention.[3,5,56,59] In the Diabetes Prevention Program, the diabetes risk reduction (vs. placebo) after ~3 years of follow-up was 31% in the metformin treatment group and 58% in the lifestyle intervention group.[3] The diabetes prevention efficacy of metformin was seen only in younger, obese (BMI >35 kg/m^2) participants, but not among older or nonobese participants.[3] In contrast, the efficacy of lifestyle intervention in preventing type 2 diabetes was uniformly observed in all age, sex, and adiposity subgroups.[3] In fact, lifestyle intervention was particularly efficacious in older Diabetes Prevention Program participants, among whom the associated decrease in incident diabetes was greater than that observed in younger participants.[64] In the Indian Diabetes Prevention Program-1, the diabetes risk reduction (vs. placebo) after 3 years of follow-up was similar in the lifestyle intervention and metformin treatment groups (28.5 and 26.4%, respectively), without evidence of an additive effect when both were tested in combination.[5] In the Indian Diabetes Prevention Program-2, a total of 407 subjects with impaired glucose tolerance (mean age 45.3 ± 6.2 years, mean BMI 25.9 ± 3.3 kg/m^2) were assigned to receive either lifestyle modification plus pioglitazone treatment (N = 204) or lifestyle modification plus placebo treatment (N = 203) and were followed for 3 years for the primary outcome of type 2 diabetes. At the end of the follow-up period, the cumulative incidence of diabetes was 29.8% in the lifestyle modification plus pioglitazone arm and 31.6% in the lifestyle modification plus placebo arm (unadjusted hazard ratio 1.084 [95% CI 0.753–1.560], P = 0.665). The Indian Diabetes Prevention Program -2 investigators reported that two subjects died and two others were hospitalized for cardiac problems in the lifestyle modification plus pioglitazone group, compared with two occurrences of cardiac disease and no death in the lifestyle modification plus placebo group.[56] Thus, the addition of pioglitazone to lifestyle modification did not significantly decrease the risk of progression from prediabetes to type 2 diabetes beyond what was achieved with lifestyle modification.[56] The SCALE study compared the effects of the glucagon-like peptide 1 (GLP-1) receptor agonist liraglutide (3 mg daily) plus lifestyle modification versus placebo plus lifestyle modification (control) on incident type 2 diabetes during 3 years of follow-up in 2,254 obese participants with prediabetes.[59] Compared with the placebo plus lifestyle modification group, the liraglutide plus lifestyle modification group showed a greater weight loss and a 79% relative risk reduction in time to diagnosis of type 2 diabetes (odds ratio 0.21 [95% CI 0.13–0.34]).[59]

Limitations of medications

In summary, the medications that have been tested for prevention of diabetes have shown efficacies that were of the same (e.g., thiazolidinediones) or lower (acarbose, metformin, or orlistat) magnitude as lifestyle modification. The occurrence of adverse effects (sometimes severe) and the need for continuous therapy to maintain their efficacy are strong reasons against the use of medications as the primary approach to diabetes prevention. The rapid glycemic rebound observed after withdrawing drugs indicates that the medications tested so far do not improve the underlying pathophysiology of prediabetes.[60–62] Moreover, when medications were tested as add-ons to lifestyle modification in two Indian trials, no additive effect was seen on reduction of diabetes risk beyond that resulting from lifestyle modification alone.[5,56] Furthermore, the cumulative costs of long-term (probably lifelong) medications (even where generic versions are available) would be burdensome in low- and middle-income countries.[65,66] Based on the foregoing realities, the use of drugs for diabetes prevention cannot be recommended as a first-line approach for the general population. Such a position is not aimed at denying a societal expectation of safe and effective medications for diabetes prevention, an acknowledgement of the limitations of currently available drug options.

Our collective poor human record of long-term adherence to dietary and exercise recommendations is compounded by physiological adaptations to weight loss that induce weight regain.[67] The quest for the ideal drug for diabetes prevention should be guided by the attributes listed in Table 7.4. Besides being well tolerated and free of adverse or toxic effects, such a medication must match or significantly exceed the magnitude of diabetes risk reduction achievable with lifestyle

Table 7.4—Characteristics of an Ideal Drug for Diabetes Prevention

- Mechanism(s): Must address key pathophysiological defects underlying prediabetes
- Regression potential: Must induce reversal of prediabetes and normalize glucose metabolism
- Durability: Should have a durable effect beyond period of exposure
- Weight: Should at least be weight neutral or preferably induce weight loss
- Safety: Must be nontoxic; use should not require safety monitoring
- Route and tolerability: Oral route preferred; must be well tolerated, without significant adverse effects
- Affordability: Should cost about the same or less than the least expensive drug for diabetes treatment

modification.[66,68,69] Most importantly, the ideal drug for diabetes prevention should have the capability of ameliorating key components of the pathophysiological defects that underlie the prediabetes state. If those defects are sufficiently repaired and normal glucoregulatory function is restored, the beneficial effects of diabetes prevention observed during drug treatment should endure and outlast the period of medication, such that cessation of drug therapy should not cause glycemic rebound. Given the ~90 million adults with prediabetes in the United States (~400 million worldwide), the ideal medication(s) for diabetes prevention should be inexpensive and must be accessible to all people at risk.

As discussed in the section addressing pathophysiology, insulin secretory compensation for ambient insulin resistance is a dominant mechanism for maintaining normoglycemia. Indeed, "insulin secretion in amounts commensurate with demand guarantees freedom from diabetes."[70] Thus, the biological effects of an ideal drug for diabetes prevention should include preservation and augmentation of pancreatic islet β-cell mass and function, through enhanced proliferation, neogenesis, anti-apoptosis, trans-differentiation of endoderm-derived cells into insulin-making cells, or other cognate mechanisms that ensure islet survival. An impact on insulin resistance, either through weight loss or independently, would also be a desirable drug attribute.

The discovery of pharmaceutical agents with the above desirable properties could usher in a new era for diabetes prevention. With such novel tools, it is conceivable that people with prediabetes who do not respond to lifestyle intervention can receive drug treatment for a defined period (e.g., 3–6 months), followed by drug withdrawal, without the risk of glycemic rebound, since the prior drug treatment would have "fixed" the underlying biological problems. If follow-up evaluation indicates early signs of dysglycemia, the regimen can be repeated ("booster"). Currently, such a pharmacologically based "vaccination" model (with possible "booster" regimens) for diabetes prevention does not exist. None of the available drugs today meet the desirable properties of the ideal diabetes prevention drug. However, it may be possible to design such a drug (or "polypill") with most of the desirable properties. A drug regimen that can improve insulin sensitivity directly and/or through induction of significant weight loss, while also improving β-cell function (perhaps through reversal of islet lipotoxicity, cell repair, regulated cellular growth, anti-apoptosis, transdifferentiation, or other means) could have a lasting diabetes prevention effect. The design of future drugs should take into account these desirable properties.

Current Guidelines for Use of Medication for Diabetes Prevention

Despite the caveats surrounding the use of medications for diabetes prevention, including the absence of any U.S. Food and Drug Administration-approved drug for such a purpose, some organizations have issued guidelines on when medications may be considered in people with prediabetes. The American Diabetes Association (ADA) consensus statement[71] and guidelines[72] rightly emphasize lifestyle modification with a weight loss goal of 5–10% as primary intervention in people with impaired fasting glucose or impaired glucose tolerance. The ADA guidelines also suggest that metformin may be considered as an adjunct to diet and exercise for the prevention of type 2 diabetes in selected high-risk individuals.[71,72] Based on the subgroup analysis of the efficacy of metformin in the Diabetes Prevention Program, metformin was most effective in preventing diabetes in very obese (BMI >35 kg/m^2) prediabetic subjects younger than 60 years of age.[3] Additional factors in favor of adjunctive treatment with metformin for diabetes prevention include a strong family history of diabetes (first-degree relatives), history of gestational diabetes, comorbid hypertension, and dyslipidemia (fasting triglycerides >150 mg/dL; HDL cholesterol levels <40 mg/dL in men and <50 mg/dL in women).[71,72] It must be noted that these recommendations regarding use of metformin are empirical; metformin was less efficacious than lifestyle intervention in the Diabetes Prevention Program, and its effect on diabetes prevention was not additive to that of lifestyle modification in the Indian Diabetes Prevention Program-1.[5] Thus, it is prudent to strive for optimal lifestyle modification at levels that have been proven to be effective (5–7% weight loss, ~700 kcal/day reduction, 150 min moderate-intensity physical activity), even in high-risk people who harbor all or most of the "indications" for metformin therapy. Whenever feasible, lifestyle modification must be the primary intervention; metformin can be considered for individuals who fail to make significant progress after reasonable exposure to lifestyle intervention. Individuals with limited mobility and those who gained weight and developed prediabetes following neuromuscular disease or spinal cord injury deserve special consideration. A primary focus on physical activity would be inappropriate or impractical in such settings, leaving dietary modification and metformin therapy as attractive options.

The guidelines regarding when to start metformin and what doses to prescribe and for how long are currently unclear. The Diabetes Prevention Program prescribed a maximum dose (1,700 mg/day [850 mg twice daily]) of immediate-release metformin, but 16% of participants took only half of that dose because of gastrointestinal symptoms.[3] Slow-release metformin formulations appear to have fewer gastrointestinal adverse effects, but those options were not explored in the Diabetes Prevention Program. In the Indian Diabetes Prevention Program-1, metformin was initiated at a dose of 250 mg twice daily and increased to 500 mg twice daily in the first 50 patients after 2 weeks. However, because of a surprisingly high frequency of hypoglycemic symptoms on the higher dose, all participants in the metformin and metformin plus lifestyle modification arms of the Indian Diabetes Prevention Program-1 were treated with 250 mg twice daily throughout the study. The median period of exposure of participants to the higher 500-mg twice-daily dose of metformin before stepping down to the lower dose was 40 days.[5] Although direct comparison is hampered by demographic, geographical, and methodological differences, the risk reduction with metformin in the U.S.-based Diabetes Prevention Program and the Indian Diabetes Prevention Program-1 (31 and 26.4%, respectively) was comparable, despite the much lower doses used in India and the lower mean BMI at enrollment of the Indian Diabetes Prevention Program-1 cohort compared with Diabetes Prevention Program participants (25.8 ± 3.5 vs. 34.0 ± 6.7 kg/m^2).[3,5] As previously noted, the magnitude of diabetes risk reduction with metformin was greater among obese Diabetes Prevention Program participants than leaner subjects.[3]

If the optimal timing of introducing metformin for diabetes prevention is to be triggered by evidence of failure of lifestyle intervention, that time can be determined empirically. In the Diabetes Prevention Program, participants assigned to lifestyle intervention lost ~7% of their initial body weight during the first 6 months. Thus, one "rule of thumb" might be a weight loss goal of 1% per month during the initial 3–6 months of lifestyle modification. Obese or overweight individuals with prediabetes who are unable to meet the monthly weight loss target of 1% after 3–6 months of lifestyle intervention would seem to be appropriate candidates for adjunctive treatment with metformin. Such an approach would be consistent with observations from behavioral weight loss studies that identify early weight loss as a strong predictor of long-term success.[73,74] Although the exact mechanisms for that observation are unclear, it is likely that early weight loss might be a marker of a highly motivated, adherent behavioral phenotype. Alternatively, it is also plausible that genetic and physiological factors (including adaptations in energy expenditure and neurohormonal signals in response to caloric restriction) may underlie individual variability in the velocity of weight loss.[75,76] Clearly, early recognition of individuals with suboptimal response to behavioral weight loss interventions would enable timely intensification of the treatment regimen. Such intensification could include motivational interviewing, increased contact frequency, enhanced self-monitoring (including self-weighing), meal substitution, and medication, among others.[77]

The prediabetes management guidelines issued by the Indian Health Services and the Australian Diabetes Society/Australian Diabetes Educators Association also emphasize lifestyle intervention, with judicious use of medications.[78,79] Per the Australian guidelines, lifestyle intervention should be tried for at least 6 months before considering medication.[79] The Indian Health Services guidelines recommend an individualized approach to the use of medication (either metformin or pioglitazone) if response to lifestyle intervention is suboptimal.[78]

Another approach to clinical decision-making regarding the use of medication for diabetes prevention is based on classification of the prediabetes state. Prediabetes is diagnosed if there is evidence of isolated impaired fasting glucose, isolated impaired glucose tolerance, or both impaired fasting glucose and impaired glucose tolerance. Individuals who have both impaired fasting glucose and impaired glucose tolerance ("double prediabetes") show more severe insulin resistance and impairment of β-cell function than individuals with a single prediabetes marker.[71,75,80] Approximately 96% of people with combined impaired fasting glucose and impaired glucose tolerance would qualify for metformin therapy, based on the ADA consensus criteria.[71,81] By contrast, only ~30% of individuals with isolated impaired fasting glucose would require metformin treatment by the same criteria. Thus, comprehensive risk stratification and rational decision-making in diabetes prevention practice would require routine assessment with an oral glucose tolerance test. The fasting plasma glucose and 2-h plasma glucose values obtained during an oral glucose tolerance test can identify individuals with isolated impaired fasting glucose, isolated impaired glucose tolerance, and the higher-risk "double prediabetes" (impaired fasting glucose plus impaired glucose tolerance) status. The latter can then be triaged to adjunctive metformin treatment.[70,75] Indeed, the ADA consensus statement recommends that the presence of both impaired fasting glucose and impaired glucose tolerance be documented if metformin is to be used for diabetes prevention.[71,72]

References

1. Eriksson KF, Lindgarde F. Prevention of type 2 (non-insulin-dependent) diabetes mellitus by diet and physical exercise: the 6-year Malmö Feasibility Study. *Diabetologia* 1991;34:891–898
2. Pan XR, Li GW, Hu YH, et al. Effects of diet and exercise in preventing NIDDM in people with impaired glucose tolerance: the Da Qing IGT and Diabetes Study. *Diabetes Care* 1997;20:537–544
3. Knowler WC, Barret-Connor E, Fowler SE, et al.; Diabetes Prevention Program Research Group. Reduction in the incidence of type 2 diabetes with lifestyle intervention or metformin. *N Engl J Med* 2002;346:393–403
4. Tuomilehto J, Lindström J, Eriksson JG, et al. Prevention of type 2 diabetes mellitus by changes in lifestyle among subjects with impaired glucose tolerance. *N Engl J Med* 2001;344:1343–1350
5. Ramachandran A, Snehalatha C, Mary S, et al. The Indian Diabetes Prevention Program shows that lifestyle modification and metformin prevent type 2 diabetes in Asian Indian subjects with impaired glucose tolerance (IDPP-1). *Diabetologia* 2006;49:289–297
6. Lindström J, Peltonen M, Eriksson JG, et al.; Finnish Diabetes Prevention Study (DPS). Improved lifestyle and decreased diabetes risk over 13 years: long-term follow-up of the randomised Finnish Diabetes Prevention Study (DPS). *Diabetologia* 2013;56:284–293

7. Gong Q, Gregg EW, Wang J, et al. Long-term effects of a randomised trial of a 6-year lifestyle intervention in impaired glucose tolerance on diabetes-related microvascular complications: the China Da Qing Diabetes Prevention Outcome Study. *Diabetologia* 2011;54:300–307
8. Diabetes Prevention Program Research Group. Long-term effects of lifestyle intervention or metformin on diabetes development and microvascular complications over 15-year follow-up: the Diabetes Prevention Program Outcomes Study. *Lancet Diabetes Endocrinol* 2015;3:866–875
9. Li G, Zhang P, Wang J, et al. The long-term effect of lifestyle interventions to prevent diabetes in the China Da Qing Diabetes Prevention Study: a 20-year follow-up study. *Lancet* 2008;371:1783–1789
10. Li G, Zhang P, Wang J, et al. Cardiovascular mortality, all-cause mortality, and diabetes incidence after lifestyle intervention for people with impaired glucose tolerance in the Da Qing Diabetes Prevention Study: a 23-year follow-up study. *Lancet Diabetes Endocrinol* 2014;2:474–480
11. Gong Q, Zhang P, Wang J, et al.; DaQing Diabetes Prevention Study Group. Morbidity and mortality after lifestyle intervention for people with impaired glucose tolerance: 30 year results of the Da Qing Diabetes Prevention Outcome Study. *Lancet Diabetes Endocrinol* 2019;7:452–461
12. Dagogo-Jack S. Prevention begets prevention: lessons from the Da Qing Study. *Nat Rev Endocrinol* 2019;15:442–443
13. Uusitupa M, Peltonen M, Lindstrom J, et al. Ten-year mortality and cardiovascular morbidity in the Finnish Diabetes Prevention Study: secondary analysis of the randomized trial. *PLoS One* 2009;4:e5656
14. Orchard TJ, Temprosa M, Goldberg R, et al. The effect of metformin and intensive lifestyle intervention on the metabolic syndrome: the Diabetes Prevention Program randomized trial. *Ann Intern Med* 2005;142:611–619
15. Ratner R, Goldberg R, Haffner S, et al. Impact of intensive lifestyle and metformin therapy on cardiovascular disease risk factors in the Diabetes Prevention Program. *Diabetes Care* 2005;28:888–894
16. Dagogo-Jack S. Primary prevention of cardiovascular disease in prediabetes: the glass is half-full and half-empty (Editorial). *Diabetes Care* 2005;28:971–972
17. Chou R, Dana T, Blazina I, et al. Statins for prevention of cardiovascular disease in adults. *JAMA* 2016;316:2008–2024
18. Terry T, Raravikar K, Chokrungvaranon N, Reaven PD. Does aggressive glycemic control benefit macrovascular and microvascular disease in type 2 diabetes? Insights from ACCORD, ADVANCE, and VADT. *Curr Cardiol Rep* 2012;14:79–88

19. Miyatake N, Wada J, Kawasaki Y, et al. Relationship between metabolic syndrome and cigarette smoking in the Japanese population. *Intern Med* 2006;45:1039–1043
20. Facchini FS, Hollenbeck CB, Jeppesen J, et al. Insulin resistance and cigarette smoking. *Lancet* 1992;339:1128–1130
21. Heizer T, Yla-Herttuala S, Luoma J, et al. Cigarette smoking potentiates endothelial dysfunction of forearm resistance vessels in patients with hypercholesterolemia: role of oxidized LDL. *Circulation* 1996;9: 1346–1353
22. Prospective Diabetes Study Group. Tight blood pressure control and risk of macrovascular and microvascular complications in type 2 diabetes: UKPDS 38. UK Prospective Diabetes Study Group. *BMJ* 1998;317: 703–713
23. McAuley PA, Artero EG, Sui X, et al. Fitness, fatness, and survival in adults with prediabetes. *Diabetes Care* 2014;37:529–536
24. Johnson JL, Slentz CA, Ross LM, et al. Ten-year legacy effects of three eight-month exercise training programs on cardiometabolic health parameters. *Front Physiol* 2019;10:452
25. Kaufman FR. Type 2 diabetes mellitus in children and youth: a new epidemic. *J Pediatr Endocrinol Metab* 2002;15(Suppl. 2):737–744
26. Duncan GE. Prevalence of diabetes and impaired fasting glucose levels among US adolescents: National Health and Nutrition Examination Survey, 1999–2002. *Arch Pediatr Adolesc Med* 2006;160:523–528
27. Pohl JH, Greer JA, Hasan KS. Type 2 diabetes mellitus in children. *Endocr Pract* 1998;4:413–416
28. Dileepan K, Feldt MM. Type 2 diabetes mellitus in children and adolescents. *Pediatr Rev* 2013;34:541–548
29. Alberti G, Zimmet P, Shaw J, et al.; Consensus Workshop Group. Type 2 diabetes in the young: the evolving epidemic: the International Diabetes Federation Consensus Workshop. *Diabetes Care* 2004;27:1798–1811
30. Wiegand S, Maikowski U, Blankenstein O, et al. Type 2 diabetes and impaired glucose tolerance in European children and adolescents with obesity: a problem that is no longer restricted to minority groups. *Eur J Endocrinol* 2004;151:199–206
31. National Institute of Diabetes and Digestive and Kidney Diseases (NIDDK). Studies to Treat or Prevent Pediatric Type 2 Diabetes (STOPP-T2D). Available from https://grants.nih.gov/grants/guide/notice-files/NOT-DK-03-006.html. Accessed 31 January 2020
32. Foster GD, Linder B, Baranowski T, et al.; HEALTHY Study Group. A school-based intervention for diabetes risk reduction. *N Engl J Med* 2010;363:443–453

33. Parsons HM. What Happened at Hawthorne? New evidence suggests the Hawthorne effect resulted from operant reinforcement contingencies. *Science* 1974;183:922–932
34. Cizza G, Piaggi P, Rother KI, Csako G; Sleep Extension Study Group. Hawthorne effect with transient behavioral and biochemical changes in a randomized controlled sleep extension trial of chronically short-sleeping obese adults: implications for the design and interpretation of clinical studies. *PLoS One* 2014;9:e104176
35. McCambridge J, Witton J, Elbourne DR. Systematic review of the Hawthorne effect: new concepts are needed to study research participation effects. *J Clin Epidemiol* 2014;3:267–277
36. Uusitupa M, Lindi V, Louheranta A, et al.; Finnish Diabetes Prevention Study Group. Long-term improvement in insulin sensitivity by changing lifestyles of people with impaired glucose tolerance: 4-year results from the Finnish Diabetes Prevention Study. *Diabetes* 2003;52:2532–2538
37. Kitabchi AE, Temprosa M, Knowler WC, et al.; Diabetes Prevention Program Research Group. Role of insulin secretion and sensitivity in the evolution of type 2 diabetes in the Diabetes Prevention Program: effects of lifestyle intervention and metformin. *Diabetes* 2005;54:2404–2414
38. Hamman RF, Wing RR, Edelstein SL, et al. Effect of weight loss with lifestyle intervention on risk of diabetes. *Diabetes Care* 2006;29:2102–2107
39. Haffner S, Temprosa M, Crandall J, et al.; Diabetes Prevention Program Research Group. Intensive lifestyle intervention or metformin on inflammation and coagulation in participants with impaired glucose tolerance. *Diabetes* 2005;54:1566–1572
40. Mather KJ, Funahashi T, Matsuzawa Y, et al.; Diabetes Prevention Program. Adiponectin, change in adiponectin, and progression to diabetes in the Diabetes Prevention Program. *Diabetes* 2008;57:980–986
41. Fulcher GR, Jones IR, Alberti KG. Improvement in glucose tolerance by reduction of lipid concentrations in non-insulin dependent diabetes mellitus. *Diabetes News* 1988;9:4–8
42. Laferrère B, Reilly D, Arias S, et al. Differential metabolic impact of gastric bypass surgery versus dietary intervention in obese diabetic subjects despite identical weight loss. *Sci Transl Med* 2011;3:80re2
43. Zhu H, Leung SW. Identification of microRNA biomarkers in type 2 diabetes: a meta-analysis of controlled profiling studies. *Diabetologia* 2015;58:900–911
44. McCaffery JM, Jablonski KA, Franks PW, et al.; Diabetes Prevention Program Research Group. *TCF7L2* polymorphism, weight loss and proinsulin:insulin ratio in the Diabetes Prevention Program. *PLoS One* 2011;6:e21518

45. Kubaszek A, Pihlajamaki J, Komarovski V, et al.; Finnish Diabetes Prevention Study. Promoter polymorphisms of the TNF-alpha (G-308A) and IL-6 (C-174G) genes predict the conversion from impaired glucose tolerance to type 2 diabetes: the Finnish Diabetes Prevention Study. *Diabetes* 2003;52:1872–1876
46. Florez JC, Jablonski KA, Sun MW, et al.; Diabetes Prevention Program Research Group. Effects of the type 2 diabetes-associated PPARG P12A polymorphism on progression to diabetes and response to troglitazone. *J Clin Endocrinol Metab* 2007;92:1502–1509
47. Diabetes Prevention Program Research Group. The Pro12Ala variant at the peroxisome proliferator-activated receptor gamma gene and change in obesity-related traits in the Diabetes Prevention Program. *Diabetologia* 2007;50:2451–2460
48. Florez JC, Jablonski KA, Bayley N, et al.; Diabetes Prevention Program Research Group. *TCF7L2* polymorphisms and progression to diabetes in the Diabetes Prevention Program. *N Engl J Med* 2006;355:241–250
49. Moore AF, Jablonski KA, Mason CC, et al.; Diabetes Prevention Program Research Group. The association of ENPP1 K121Q with diabetes incidence is abolished by lifestyle modification in the Diabetes Prevention Program. *J Clin Endocrinol Metab* 2009;94:449–455
50. Ackermann RT, Marrero DG. Adapting the Diabetes Prevention Program lifestyle intervention for delivery in the community: the YMCA model. *Diabetes Educ* 2007;33:69,74–75,77–78
51. Albright AL, Gregg EW. Preventing type 2 diabetes in communities across the U.S.: the National Diabetes Prevention Program. *Am J Prev Med* 2013;44(4 Suppl. 4):S346–S351
52. Chiasson JL, Josse RG, Gomis R, et al. STOP-NIDDM Trial Research Group. Acarbose for prevention of type 2 diabetes mellitus: the STOP-NIDDM randomized trial. *Lancet* 2002;359:2072–2077
53. Torgerson JS, Hauptman J, Boldrin MN, Sjostrom L. XENical in the prevention of diabetes in obese subjects (XENDOS) study: a randomized study of orlistat as an adjunct to lifestyle changes for the prevention of type 2 diabetes in obese patients. *Diabetes Care* 2004;27:155–161
54. The DREAM (Diabetes Reduction Assessment with Ramipril and Rosiglitazone Medication) Trial Investigators. Effect of rosiglitazone on the frequency of diabetes in patients with impaired glucose tolerance or impaired fasting glucose: a randomized controlled trial. *Lancet* 2006;368:1096–1105
55. DeFronzo RA, Tripathy D, Schwenke DC, et al.; ACT NOW Study. Pioglitazone for diabetes prevention in impaired glucose tolerance. *N Engl J Med* 2011;364:1104–1115

56. Ramachandran A, Snehalatha C, Mary S, et al. Pioglitazone does not enhance the effectiveness of lifestyle modification in preventing conversion of impaired glucose tolerance to diabetes in Asian Indians: results of the Indian Diabetes Prevention Program-2 (IDPP-2). *Diabetologia* 2009;52:1019–1026
57. Zinman B, Stewart BH, Neuman J, et al. Low-dose combination therapy with rosiglitazone and metformin to prevent type 2 diabetes mellitus (CANOE trial): a double-blind randomized controlled study. *Lancet* 2010;376:103–111
58. NAVIGATOR Study Group. Effect of valsartan on the incidence of diabetes and cardiovascular events. *N Engl J Med* 2010;362:1477–1490
59. Le Roux CW, Astrup A, Fujioka K, et al.; SCALE Obesity Prediabetes NN8022-1839 Study Group. 3 Years of liraglutide versus placebo for type 2 diabetes risk reduction and weight management in individuals with prediabetes: a randomized, double-blind trial. *Lancet* 2017;389:1399–1409
60. Diabetes Prevention Program Research Group. Effects of withdrawal from metformin on the development of diabetes in the Diabetes Prevention Program. *Diabetes Care* 2003;26:977–980
61. DREAM Trial Investigators. Incidence of diabetes following ramipril or rosiglitazone withdrawal. *Diabetes Care* 2011;34:1265–1269
62. Tripathy D, Schwenke DC, Banerji M, et al. Diabetes incidence and glucose tolerance after termination of pioglitazone therapy: results from ACT NOW. *J Clin Endocrinol Metab* 2016;101:2056–2062
63. Pi-Sunyer X, Astrup A, Fujioka K, et al.; SCALE Obesity and Prediabetes NN8022-1839 Study Group. A randomized, controlled trial of 3.0 mg of liraglutide in weight management. *N Engl J Med* 2015;373:11–22
64. Crandall J, Schade D, Ma Y, et al.; Diabetes Prevention Program Research Group. The influence of age on the effects of lifestyle modification and metformin in prevention of diabetes. *J Gerontol A Biol Sci Med Sci* 2006; 61:1075–1081
65. Diabetes Prevention Program Research Group. The 10-year cost-effectiveness of lifestyle intervention or metformin for diabetes prevention: an intent-to-treat analysis of the DPP/DPPOS. *Diabetes Care* 2012;35: 723–730
66. Echouffo-Tcheugui JB, Dagogo-Jack S. Preventing diabetes mellitus in developing countries. *Nat Rev Endocrinol* 2012;8:557–562
67. Greenway FL. Physiological adaptations to weight loss and factors favouring weight regain. *Int J Obes (Lond)* 2015;39:1188–1196
68. Pour OR, Dagogo-Jack S. Prediabetes as a therapeutic target. *Clin Chem* 2011;57:215–220

69. Nyenwe EA, Dagogo-Jack S. Metabolic syndrome, prediabetes and the science of primary prevention. *Minerva Endocrinol* 2011;36:129–145
70. Dagogo-Jack S. 2015 Presidential address: 75 years of battling diabetes: our global challenge. *Diabetes Care* 2016;39:3–9
71. Nathan DM, Davidson MB, DeFronzo RA, et al. Impaired fasting glucose and impaired glucose tolerance. *Diabetes Care* 2007;30:753–759
72. American Diabetes Association. 3. Prevention or delay of type 2 diabetes: *Standards of Medical Care in Diabetes—2020. Diabetes Care* 2020;43: S32–S36
73. Gow ML, Baur LA, Ho M, et al. Can early weight loss, eating behaviors and socioeconomic factors predict successful weight loss at 12- and 24-months in adolescents with obesity and insulin resistance participating in a randomised controlled trial? *Int J Behav Nutr Phys Act* 2016;13:43
74. Feig EH, Lowe MR. Variability in weight change early in behavioral weight loss treatment: theoretical and clinical implications. *Obesity* 2017;25: 1509–1515
75. Dagogo-Jack S. Physiological and hormonal factors that influence leptin production. In *Leptin: Regulation and Clinical Applications.* 1st ed. Dagogo-Jack S, Ed. New York, Springer, 2015, pp. 45–66
76. Page-Wilson G, Dagogo-Jack S. Central and peripheral modulators of appetite and satiety. In *Nutrition and Diabetes.* 2nd ed. Opara E, Dagogo-Jack S, Eds. Boca Raton, FL, CRC Press, 2019, pp. 3–26
77. Dagogo-Jack S, Egbuonu N, Edeoga C. Principles and practice of non-pharmacological interventions to reduce cardiometabolic risk. *Med Princ Pract* 2010;19:167–175
78. Indian Health Services. IHS guidelines for care of adults with prediabetes and/or the metabolic syndrome in clinical settings, 2008. Available from http://aianp.ucdenver.edu/sdpi/common/initiative/DP_Appendices/DPIAN6%20IHS%20Guidelines%20PreDiabetes%20Metsyn%20Sept%20 2008.pdf. Accessed 30 January 2020
79. Twigg SM, Kamp MC, Davis TM, et al.; Australian Diabetes Society and Australian Diabetes Educators Association. Prediabetes: a position statement from the Australian Diabetes Society and Australian Diabetes Educators Association. *Med J Aust* 2007;186:461–465
80. Kanat M, Mari A, Norton L, et al. Distinct β-cell defects in impaired fasting glucose and impaired glucose tolerance. *Diabetes* 2012;61:447–453
81. Rhee MK, Herrick K, Ziemer DC, et al. Many Americans have prediabetes and should be considered for metformin therapy. *Diabetes Care* 2010;33:49–54

Chapter 8

Reversal of Prediabetes and Restoration of Normal Glucose Regulation

Without intervention, most people with prediabetes will develop type 2 diabetes. Long-term observational follow-up of participants in the Whitehall II study showed that most people with A1C-defined prediabetes had persistent prediabetes or progressed to type 2 diabetes during 5 years of follow-up.[1]

In the Da Qing study, the cumulative 30-year incidence of type 2 diabetes was ~96% among participants assigned to the control group.[2] However, during shorter-term follow-up, many individuals will have persistent prediabetes and some may even revert to normal glucose regulation.[1,3] Diabetes prevention studies have focused mostly on preventing or delaying the progression from prediabetes to type 2 diabetes. Among individuals in whom type 2 diabetes was successfully prevented by intervention, persistent prediabetes is a more frequent end-state than reversion to normal glucose regulation.[1–3] Individuals with persistent prediabetes are at increased risks of developing serious vascular complications. Thus, persistence of the prediabetes state represents a suboptimal response to interventions, although such an outcome is still better than progression to type 2 diabetes. However, it is more desirable for the focus of intervention to shift from prevention of type 2 diabetes to regression of the prediabetes state and restoration of normal glucose regulation. What follows is a review of clinical trials that have reported data on the regression of prediabetes. There are numerous advantages associated with restoration of normal glucose regulation in people with prediabetes.

Lifetyle-Mediated Regression of Prediabetes

Several randomized controlled trials, using lifestyle intervention for diabetes prevention, have provided information on the proportion of participants who experienced regression of prediabetes and achieved restoration of normal glucose regulation status[4–15] (Table 8.1).

Table 8.1—Reversal of Prediabetes in Randomized Controlled Trials Using Lifestyle and/or Medication Interventions

Study	Duration (years)	Interventions	Reversal of Prediabetes
Malmö study[4]	6	Lifestyle vs. placebo	52.2%
DPP[3,7]	2.8	Lifestyle vs. metformin vs. placebo	Lifestyle 40% Metformin 20% Placebo 20%
STOP-NIDDM[8]	3.3	Acarbose vs. placebo	35%
DREAM[9,10]	3	Rosiglitazone vs. placebo	50.5%
ACT NOW[11,12]	2.4	Pioglitazone vs. placebo	48%

ACT NOW, Actos Now for the Prevention of Diabetes; DPP, Diabetes Prevention Program; DREAM, Diabetes Reduction Assessment with Ramipril and Rosiglitazone Medication; STOP-NIDDM, Study to Prevent Non-Insulin-Dependent Diabetes Mellitus.

Malmö study

The Malmö study investigators enrolled and randomized Swedish men with impaired glucose tolerance ($N = 181$) or early-stage type 2 diabetes ($N = 41$) to a lifestyle intervention group or a control group.[4] The lifestyle group received supervised physical activity training for 60 minutes twice weekly for 6 months along with dietary counseling. The lifestyle intervention recipients lost ~3.7% of body weight, whereas body weight in the comparison group (subjects with impaired glucose tolerance who did not receive the lifestyle intervention) increased by ~1.7% during the intervention.[4] Assessment after ~6 years of follow-up indicated that 52.2% of participants with impaired glucose tolerance in the intervention group had reverted to normal glucose tolerance with lifestyle modification.[4] The glycemic improvements were accompanied by tandem improvements in blood pressure, lipids, and hyperinsulinemia.[4] Furthermore, the investigators observed restoration of acute insulin secretory response to glucose associated with regression of prediabetes.[4]

Diabetes Prevention Program

After 2.8 years of follow-up in the Diabetes Prevention Program, ~40% of participants randomized to the intensive lifestyle modification arm achieved normal glucose regulation versus ~20% in the metformin arm and ~20% in the placebo arm.[3,5] The predictors of regression of prediabetes among Diabetes Prevention Program participants included greater weight loss, lower baseline fasting plasma glucose, and 2-h plasma glucose values, younger age, and insulin secretory response.[5] Family history of diabetes, lipid profiles, blood pressure, use of medications (antihypertensives, lipid-lowering drugs, hormone replacement), dietary fat calories, and physical activity were not significant predictors of regression to normal glucose regulation in the Diabetes Prevention Program.[5] A follow-up analysis considered adherence to Diabetes Prevention Program interventions and risk stratification for diabetes.[16] Among participants at lowest risk of developing diabetes, those who adhered to lifestyle intervention had an 8% absolute risk reduction of developing diabetes and a 35% greater absolute likelihood of reverting to normal glucose regulation compared with placebo-adherent participants.[16] Among participants at highest risk of developing diabetes, those who adhered to lifestyle intervention had a 39% absolute risk reduction of developing diabetes and a 24% greater absolute likelihood of reverting to normal glucose regulation compared with placebo-adherent subjects.[16] Adherence to lifestyle intervention was defined as achieving a weight loss >5% of initial weight by the 6-month visit.[16] These analyses showed that weight loss is a significant mechanism for regression of prediabetes in people at either lower or higher risk for diabetes. Compared with lifestyle intervention, the findings regarding adherence to metformin indicated lower magnitudes of benefits regarding prevention of diabetes or regression of prediabetes in both participants at low or high risk of developing diabetes. Adherence to metformin intervention among participants at lowest risk of developing diabetes resulted in no reduction in their risk of developing diabetes but was associated with a 17% greater absolute likelihood of reverting to normal glucose regulation.[16] Among participants at highest risk of developing diabetes, those who adhered to metformin intervention had a 25% absolute risk reduction of developing diabetes and an 11% greater absolute likelihood of reverting to normal glucose regulation compared with placebo-adherent subjects.[16]

Interestingly, assignment to intensive lifestyle intervention, independent of weight loss, predicted regression of prediabetes and restoration of normal glucose regulation. However, caloric intake and MET-hours per week of physical activity were specifically examined and found not to be independent predictors of regression to normal glucose regulation in the Diabetes Prevention Program cohort.[5] Thus, although weight loss was a major driver of regression, the combination of healthy eating, increased physical activity, changes in body composition (e.g., decreased visceral fat), and other pleitropic benefits of lifestyle intervention might have accounted for the reversal of prediabetes that occurred in the participants who did lose weight.[5,17,18]

Thus, both the Malmö study and Diabetes Prevention Program showed that lifestyle-based interventions used in those studies induced reversal from prediabetes and restored normal glucose regulation in some 40–50% of participants. Notably, the mean weight loss response to lifestyle intervention was ~3.7% in the Malmö study and ~4% in the Diabetes Prevention Program at the end of the initial follow-up period of ~6 and ~3 years, respectively. Thus, it is conceivable that lifestyle interventions that achieve greater weight loss could yield even greater potency on regression of prediabetes.

Drug-Induced Regression of Prediabetes

Data on regression of prediabetes are available for some pharmacological agents, tested alone or in combination with lifestyle interventions.

Acarbose

The multinational Study to Prevent Non-Insulin-Dependent Diabetes Mellitus (STOP-NIDDM) compared the effects of acarbose (100 mg three times a day) versus a placebo in participants with impaired glucose tolerance (mean age 54 years, mean BMI 31.0 kg/m^2).[8] The investigators reported that after 3 years of follow-up, 35% of participants with impaired glucose tolerance treated with acarbose had experienced regression of prediabetes and achieved normal glucose tolerance status. Unfortunately, 3 months after stopping acarbose, rebound in blood glucose occurred. Thus, the regression of prediabetes was not sustained without medication.[8]

Thiazolidinedione

Participants enrolled with impaired fasting glucose and/or impaired glucose tolerance in the DREAM (Diabetes Reduction Assessment with Ramipril and Rosiglitazone Medication) trial were randomly assigned to treatment with rosiglitazone (4 mg once daily for 2 months, then 8 mg once daily) or a placebo. After 3 years of follow-up of this middle-aged, obese cohort (mean age 55 years, mean BMI 31 kg/m^2), 50.5% of participants in the rosiglitazone arm had achieved normoglycemia compared to 30.3% in the placebo arm.[9] However, the effect of rosiglitazone waned when the drug was withdrawn.[10] The Actos Now for the Prevention of Diabetes (ACT NOW) study reported prediabetes regression data for another thiazolidinedione, pioglitazone.[11] After a median 2.4 years of follow-up of the study participants (mean age 52 years, mean BMI 34 kg/m^2), all of whom had prediabetes (impaired glucose tolerance) at baseline, regression of prediabetes and reversion to normal glucose regulation occurred in 48% of participants treated with pioglitazone and 28% of subjects treated with a placebo.[11] The drug effect on prediabetes regression was not sustained; the proportion of participants with normal glucose regulation decreased to 23% within 11 months after stopping pioglitazone.[12] In the Indian Diabetes Prevention Program-2, another trial of pioglitazone in a leaner Indian prediabetes population (mean age 45 years, mean BMI 26 kg/m^2), 40.9% of participants randomized to lifestyle modification plus pioglitazone treatment reverted to normoglycemia, compared to 32.3% randomized to lifestyle modification plus placebo treatment who reverted to normoglycemia.[19]

Fixed-dose combination of metformin and rosiglitazone

In the Diabetes Prevention Program, metformin showed no greater potency than a placebo on the outcome of prediabetes reversal and restoration of normal glucose regulation.[3] Investigators in the Canadian Normoglycemia Outcomes Evaluation (CANOE) study tested the effects of a fixed-dose combination regimen (metformin 500 mg plus rosiglitazone 2 mg taken two times daily) versus a placebo in participants with impaired glucose tolerance (mean age 52 years, mean BMI 32 kg/m^2). Regression of prediabetes and reversion to normal glucose regulation occurred in 80% of participants treated with the low-dose metformin-plus-rosiglitazone regimen, compared to 53% of participants treated with placebo who reverted to normoglycemia.[13]

Liraglutide

Although not strictly a diabetes prevention trial, the subgroup of subjects with prediabetes (N = 2,285) in a randomized controlled trial of the glucagon-like peptide 1 (GLP-1) receptor agonist liraglutide (3 mg) for obesity treatment provides some insight on regression of prediabetes.[14,15] At 56 weeks, regression of prediabetes occurred in 69% of subjects randomized to lifestyle modification plus liraglutide 3-mg treatment, compared to 36% of participants in the lifestyle modification plus placebo group.[14,15] The proportions with regression of prediabetes were sustained during 3 years of medication and lifestyle intervention (66% in the liraglutide group and 36% in the placebo group).[14] Reocurrence of prediabetes was noted after ~3 months of stopping liraglutide.[14,15] The benefits demonstrated by liraglutide are consistent with data from prior preclinical and clinical studies on the effects of treatment with dipeptidyl peptidase-4 inhibitors (which raise plasma GLP-1 levels) and GLP-1 receptor agonists in animal models and people with prediabetes.[20]

The lack of sustained effect on regression of prediabetes after stopping mediations is disappointing and quite in contrast to the sustained efficacy of lifestyle modification. Lifestyle intervention was associated with major health benefits, including decreased mortality, in Malmö study participants assessed 12 years after cessation of active intervention.[21] Similar evidence of a legacy effect of lifestyle modification was demonstrated in long-term, post-intervention follow-up studies of the Diabetes Prevention Program, the Finnish Diabetes Prevention Study, the and Da Qing study.[22–24]

Clinical Impact of Regression from Prediabetes to Normal Glucose Regulation

Besides the risk of progression to type 2 diabetes, prediabetes is a fertile ground for the initiation of microvascular and macrovascular complications.[25,26] Reversal of prediabetes should, thus, decrease the risk, not only of future diabetes, but also of developing serious prediabetic vascular complications. Further analysis of data from a continued follow-up study of the Diabetes Prevention Program participants (Diabetes Prevention Program Outcomes Study) revealed that participants who experienced regression of prediabetes and restoration of normal glucose regulation enjoyed a 56% reduction in diabetes incidence during long-term follow-up.[27] The reduction in long-term diabetes incidence in people with prediabetes who achieved normal glucose regulation was observed, even among participants whose normal glucose regulation status was unsustained and whose glucose levels later returned to prediabetes levels.[27] The number of times a participant achieved normal glucose regulation during the several years of follow-up was associated with the magnitude of future diabetes risk reduction. Participants who reached normal glucose regulation once showed a 47% reduction in future diabetes risk; individuals who achieved normal glucose regulation twice had a 61% reduction; and subjects who achieved normal glucose regulation three times were associated with a 67% reduction in long-term incidence of type 2 diabetes.[27] Thus, regression from prediabetes to normal glucose regulation, even transiently, was protective of future risk of glycemic progression to type 2 diabetes. With such a large effect on future risk of type 2 diabetes, reversal of prediabetes and restoration of normal glucose regulation should be promoted as the primary goals for intervention in people with prediabetes. Achieving regression of prediabetes and a return to normal glucose regulation would be of enormous public health benefit, since that would prevent the development of type 2 diabetes and its complications.

The latter notion is supported by the observation that the Diabetes Prevention Program participants who achieved regression of prediabetes enjoyed relative protection from developing microvascular disease during a median follow-up of 15 years.[28] Restoration of normal glucose regulation status, in previously prediabetic subjects, has also been shown to decrease the occurrence of macrovascular complications.[1,6,29]

Findings from the Whitehall II study, a long-term observational cohort, showed that reversion from 2-h plasma glucose-defined prediabetes to normoglycemia was associated with reduction of future risk of cardiovascular disease and mortality.[1] In a study of individuals with prediabetes complicated by peripheral neuropathy, a 1-year lifestyle intervention program that resulted in glycemic normalization was associated with histological recovery of neuropathy and reinnervation, as demonstrated by the measurement of intraepidermal nerve fiber density.[30]

There is now compelling evidence that the natural history of prediabetes bends toward development of type 2 diabetes or persistence of the prediabetes state, rather than spontaneous remisson. Despite the impressive efficacy of interventions in preventing type 2 diabetes among people with prediabetes, a substantial proportion (~50%) remain with persistent prediabetes.

The association of prediabetes with microvascular and macrovascular complications, not only future diabetes risk, should shift the goal of intervention in people with prediabetes from diabetes prevention to prediabetes reversal.

The experience from clinical trials suggests that the lifestyle intervention protocols were more effective in preventing progression from prediabetes to type 2 diabetes than they were at inducing regression of prediabetes. There appears to be a relationship between the amount of weight loss and degree of glycemic normalization. The Diabetes Prevention Program lifestyle participants who experienced regression from prediabetes to normal glucose regulation lost more weight than those with persistent prediabetes.[5] Parenthetically, both groups were successful at preventing progression to type 2 diabetes. However, the group who achieved glucose normalization stood to gain far more, including additional protection from a long-term risk of developing diabetes and related complications. Among Look AHEAD study participants with a short duration type 2 diabetes diagnosis (<2 years), a weight loss of >6.5% from baseline body weight was associated with remission of diabetes (defined as maintenance of A1C <6.5% without medications for at least 2–4 years).[31]

Longitudinal studies have discovered that healthy, normoglycemic individuals may experience impaired glucose regulation leading to the development initially of prediabetes and subsequently type 2 diabetes (Fig. 8.1). Because prediabetes is a risk factor for future diabetes and multiple microvascular and macrovascular complications, specific protocols for reversal of prediabetes and restoration of normal glucose regulation need to be developed and tested. The design of such protocols should be informed by available data on the relationship between weight loss and degree of glycemic normalization as well as a deeper understanding of the pathobiology (triggers, predictors, mechanism, mediators) of prediabetes summarized in the earlier sections of this book (Table 3.1).

There is heterogeneity in the weight and BMI distributions of people with prediabetes. The pathobiology of dysglycemia among individuals at the normal or nonobese range of the weight and BMI distribution needs to be better understood, to inform the design of preventive interventions. Notably, the participants with prediabetes enrolled in the Indian Diabetes Prevention Program-1 (baseline BMI 25.8 ± 3.5 kg/m^2) were not overweight by Western standards and did not lose weight at the end of 3 years of lifestyle intervention.[32] Yet, compared with the

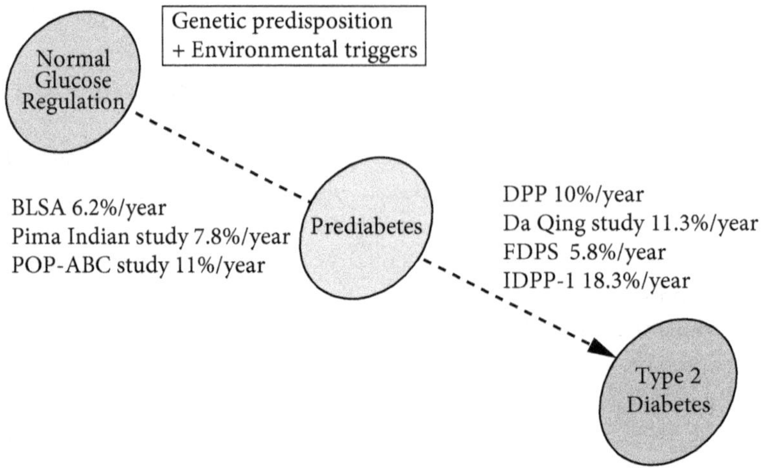

Figure 8.1—Rates of progression from normal glucose regulation to prediabetes and from prediabetes to type 2 diabetes in various longitudinal studies. BLSA, Baltimore Longitudinal Study on Aging; DPP, Diabetes Prevention Program; FDPS, Finnish Diabetes Prevention Study; IDPP-1, Indian Diabetes Prevention Program 1; POP-ABC, Pathobiology of Prediabetes in a Biracial Cohort.

control group, the incidence of diabetes was reduced by 28.5% in the lifestyle intervention group.[32] Thus, elements of the lifestyle intervention used in that study, such as dietary modification (decreased intake of refined carbohydrates and fats and increased intake of dietary fiber) and physical activity (at least 30 min daily), proved beneficial without inducing weight loss.[32] The mechanisms of such apparent weight loss–independent benefits need further elucidation. It is possible that the increased physical activity along with healthier eating patterns exerted favorable effects on fitness, body fat distribution, and/or other metabolic end points that led to the observed decrease in type 2 diabetes incidence.[33,34]

Exploitation of knowledge of the contributions of dietary habits, physical inactivity, adiposity, insulin resistance, β-cell defects, lipid moieties, inflammatory markers, metabolites, microbiome and microRNAs, and other factors to the pathogenesis of prediabetes should yield useful insights. These factors can be modeled to generate risk engines that could help predict which individuals with normal glucose regulation would break out of regulation and progress to prediabetes and who would revert from prediabetes to normal glucose regulation.[35] The increased knowledge should also aid in the design of novel, targeted interventions for the reversal of prediabetes and restoration of normal glucose regulation. The approach to the identification of at-risk populations for preventive interventions is discussed in Chapter 9 (Strategies for diabetes prevention in the community).

References

1. Vistisen D, Kivimäki M, Perreault L, et al.; Reversion from prediabetes to normoglycaemia and risk of cardiovascular disease and mortality: the Whitehall II cohort study. *Diabetologia* 2019;62:1385–1390
2. Gong Q, Zhang P, Wang J, et al.; DaQing Diabetes Prevention Study Group. Morbidity and mortality after lifestyle intervention for people with impaired glucose tolerance: 30 year results of the Da Qing Diabetes Prevention Outcome Study. *Lancet Diabetes Endocrinol* 2019;7:452–461
3. Knowler WC, Barret-Connor E, Fowler SE, et al.; Diabetes Prevention Program Research Group. Reduction in the incidence of type 2 diabetes with lifestyle intervention or metformin. *N Engl J Med* 2002;346:393–403
4. Eriksson KF, Lindgarde F. Prevention of type 2 (non-insulin-dependent) diabetes mellitus by diet and physical exercise: the 6-year Malmö feasibility study. *Diabetologia* 1991;34:891–898
5. Perreault L, Kahn SE, Christophi CA, et al.; Diabetes Prevention Program Research Group. Regression from pre-diabetes to normal glucose regulation in the Diabetes Prevention Program. *Diabetes Care* 2009;32:1583–1588
6. Sallar A, Dagogo-Jack S. Regression from prediabetes to normal glucose regulation: state of the science. *Exp Biol Med (Maywood)* 2020;24:889–896
7. Coppell K, Freer T, Abel S, et al. What predicts regression from prediabetes to normal glucose regulation following a primary care nurse-delivered dietary intervention? A study protocol for a prospective cohort study. *BMJ Open* 2019;9:e033358
8. Chiasson JL, Josse RG, Gomis R, et al. STOP-NIDDM Trial Research Group. Acarbose for prevention of type 2 diabetes mellitus: the STOP-NIDDM randomized trial. *Lancet* 2002;359:2072–2077
9. DREAM (Diabetes Reduction Assessment with Ramipril and Rosiglitazone Medication) Trial Investigators. Effect of rosiglitazone on the frequency of diabetes in patients with impaired glucose tolerance or impaired fasting glucose: a randomized controlled trial. *Lancet* 2006;368:1096–1105
10. DREAM Trial Investigators. Incidence of diabetes following ramipril or rosiglitazone withdrawal. *Diabetes Care* 2011;34:1265–1269
11. DeFronzo RA, Tripathy D, Schwenke DC, et al.; ACT NOW Study. Pioglitazone for diabetes prevention in impaired glucose tolerance. *N Engl J Med* 2011;364:1104–1115

12. Tripathy D, Schwenke DC, Banerji M, et al. Diabetes incidence and glucose tolerance after termination of pioglitazone therapy: results from ACT NOW. *J Clin Endocrinol Metab* 2016;101:2056–2062
13. Zinman B, Stewart BH, Neuman J, et al. Low-dose combination therapy with rosiglitazone and metformin to prevent type 2 diabetes mellitus (CANOE trial): a double-blind randomized controlled study. *Lancet* 2010;376:103–111
14. Pi-Sunyer X, Astrup A, Fujioka K, et al.; SCALE Obesity and Prediabetes NN8022-1839 Study Group. A randomized, controlled trial of 3.0 mg of liraglutide in weight management. *N Engl J Med* 2015;373:11–22
15. Le Roux CW, Astrup A, Fujioka K, et al.; SCALE Obesity Prediabetes NN8022-1839 Study Group. 3 Years of liraglutide versus placebo for type 2 diabetes risk reduction and weight management in individuals with prediabetes: a randomized, double-blind trial. *Lancet* 2017;389:1399–1409
16. Herman WH, Pan Q, Edelstein SL, et al.; Diabetes Prevention Program Research Group. Impact of lifestyle and metformin interventions on the risk of progression to diabetes and regression to normal glucose regulation in overweight or obese people with impaired glucose regulation. *Diabetes Care* 2017;40:1668–1677
17. Giannopoulou I, Ploutz-Snyder LL, Carhart R, et al. Exercise is required for visceral fat loss in postmenopausal women with type 2 diabetes. *J Clin Endocrinol Metab* 2005;90:1511–1518
18. Conn VS, Hafdahl AR, Mehr DR, et al. Metabolic effects of interventions to increase exercise in adults with type 2 diabetes. *Diabetologia* 2007;50: 913–921
19. Ramachandran A, Snehalatha C, Mary S, et al. Pioglitazone does not enhance the effectiveness of lifestyle modification in preventing conversion of impaired glucose tolerance to diabetes in Asian Indians: results of the Indian Diabetes Prevention Program-2 (IDDP-2). *Diabetologia* 2009;52:1019–1026
20. Papaetis GS. Incretin-based therapies in prediabetes: current evidence and future perspectives. *World J Diabetes* 2014;5:817–834
21. Eriksson KF, Lindgärde F. No excess 12-year mortality in men with impaired glucose tolerance who participated in the Malmö Preventive Trial with diet and exercise. *Diabetologia* 1998;41:1010–1016
22. Knowler WC, Fowler SE, Hamman RF, et al.; Diabetes Prevention Program Research Group. 10-Year follow-up of diabetes incidence and weight loss in the Diabetes Prevention Program Outcomes Study. *Lancet* 2009;374:1677–1686

23. Lindström J, Ilanne-Parikka P, Peltonen M, et al.; Finnish Diabetes Prevention Study Group. Sustained reduction in the incidence of type 2 diabetes by lifestyle intervention: follow-up of the Finnish Diabetes Prevention Study. *Lancet* 2006;368:1673–1679
24. Gong Q, Zhang P, Wang J, et al.; DaQing Diabetes Prevention Study Group. Morbidity and mortality after lifestyle intervention for people with impaired glucose tolerance: 30-year results of the Da Qing Diabetes Prevention Outcome Study. *Lancet Diabetes Endocrinol* 2019;7:452–461
25. Brannick B, Dagogo-Jack S. Prediabetes and cardiovascular disease pathophysiology and interventions for prevention and risk reduction. *Endocrinol Metab Clin North Am* 2018;47:33–50
26. Brannick B, Wynn A, Dagogo-Jack S. Prediabetes as a toxic environment for the initiation of microvascular and macrovascular complications. *Exp Biol Med (Maywood)* 2016;241:1323–1331
27. Perreault L, Pan Q, Mather KJ, et al.; Diabetes Prevention Program Research Group. Effect of regression from prediabetes to normal glucose regulation on long-term reduction in diabetes risk: results from the Diabetes Prevention Program Outcomes Study. *Lancet* 2012;379:2243–2251
28. Perreault L, Pan Q, Schroeder EB, et al.; Diabetes Prevention Program Research Group. Regression from prediabetes to normal glucose regulation and prevalence of microvascular disease in the Diabetes Prevention Program Outcomes Study. *Diabetes Care* 2019;42:1809–1815
29. Perreault L, Temprosa M, Mather KJ, et al.; Diabetes Prevention Program Research Group. Regression from prediabetes to normal glucose regulation is associated with reduction in cardiovascular risk: results from the Diabetes Prevention Program Outcomes Study. *Diabetes Care* 2014;37:2622–2631
30. Smith AG, Russell J, Feldman EL, et al. Lifestyle intervention for prediabetic neuropathy. *Diabetes Care* 2006;29:1294–1299
31. Gregg EW, Chen H, Wagenknecht LE, et al.; Look AHEAD Research Group. Association of an intensive lifestyle intervention with remission of type 2 diabetes. *JAMA* 2012;308:2489–2496
32. Ramachandran A, Snehalatha C, Mary S, et al. The Indian Diabetes Prevention Program shows that lifestyle modification and metformin prevent type 2 diabetes in Asian Indian subjects with impaired glucose tolerance (IDPP-1). *Diabetologia* 2006;49:289–297
33. McAuley PA, Artero EG, Sui X, et al. Fitness, fatness, and survival in adults with prediabetes. *Diabetes Care* 2014;37:529–536

34. Johnson JL, Slentz CA, Ross LM, et al. Ten-year legacy effects of three eight-month exercise training programs on cardiometabolic health parameters. *Front Physiol* 2019;10:452
35. Hwang YC, Cho IJ, Jeong IK, et al. Factors associated with regression from prediabetes to normal glucose tolerance in a Korean general population: a community-based 10-year prospective cohort study. *Diabet Med* 2018;35:1544–1551

Chapter 9

Translating Diabetes Prevention Practice in the Community

The translation of any novel remedies, research findings, or discoveries related to human health from the research arena to the community can be conceptualized within the framework of *1*) effective communication, comprehension, evaluation, and acceptance of the new ideas among a targeted translation delivery group (e.g., primary care physicians); *2*) incorporation of the new information into the core professional knowledge base and dissemination to a wider circle of professionals and learners; *3*) further diffusion of the novel message into the general populace, through education, demonstration, and practices by opinion leaders; *4*) adoption of evidence-based changes in practices and behaviors, as a result of the new knowledge; and *5*) evaluation of impact, tweaking of strategies, improvements, and promotion of best practices. The preceding construct of the translational cascade is somewhat akin to the sequential steps in Prochaska's transtheoretical model of behavior modification: precontemplative, contemplative, preparation, action (i.e., behavior change), and maintenance.[1,2]

The Diabetes Prevention Program demonstrated that ~10% of subjects with impaired glucose tolerance and high-normal fasting plasma glucose progressed to clinical diabetes each year over an average of 2.8 years of follow-up in the study.[3] The results of the Diabetes Prevention Program, the Finnish Diabetes Prevention Study, and other studies showed ~25–60% relative risk reduction for incident type 2 diabetes from lifestyle modification compared to a placebo.[3–6] In both the Diabetes Prevention Program and the Finnish Diabetes Prevention Study, every 1-kg decrease in weight in the lifestyle arm was associated with a 15–16% decrease in future type 2 diabetes risk.[3,5] The Da Qing study in China showed that lifestyle intervention not only significantly decreased progression from prediabetes to type 2 diabetes, but it also reduced the occurrence of microvascular complications, cardiovascular disease events, cardiovascular disease deaths, and all-cause mortality after 30 years of follow-up.[7] These messages need to be packaged and disseminated widely in the community.

Dissemination of Diabetes Prevention Knowledge

The preponderance of evidence from randomized clinical trials on the efficacy of lifestyle intervention in preventing type 2 diabetes has established the rationale for diabetes prevention as self-evident among health professionals. However, the screening for prediabetes has not become routine practice, even in economically advanced countries. Bridging the hiatus between philosophical acceptance of the idea of diabetes prevention among health professionals and the adoption of pragmatic steps to detect and act on high-risk individuals requires a reasoned and deliberate strategy.

The information and knowledge base of health care professionals must be nudged toward greater awareness of the burden of prediabetes and the feasibility of primary prevention of diabetes through validated approaches. Beginning with early education, curriculum development in primary and high schools should introduce pertinent information from the behavioral components of the landmark diabetes prevention studies within a wider context of wellness and health maintenance. Next, students in the health professions should be exposed to formal instruction on the design and key findings of the landmark diabetes prevention studies, again, within the wider context of wellness. Residency training programs in the clinical disciplines (particularly, family practice, internal medicine, pediatrics, and obstetrics and gynecology) should incorporate modules on diabetes prevention as part of the core curriculum lectures, further consolidated by electives in Endocrinology and Diabetes. Finally, practicing physicians in all disciplines (including internists, family physicians, endocrinologists, cardiologists, nephrologists, and general and specialist surgeons) as well as podiatrists, nurses, nurse practitioners, pharmacists, and other primary care providers must have their knowledge base updated, so they can become advocates and implementers of primary prevention of diabetes.

Increased awareness of the feasibility of preventing type 2 diabetes among primary care providers and the general medical community should induce enthusiasm for the screening and detection of individuals with prediabetes (usually relatives of patients with established type 2 diabetes as well as overweight, obese, or habitually sedentary individuals). The current rate of screening and documentation of prediabetes status is abysmal, since most people with prediabetes in the general population remain undiagnosed and unaware of their condition.[8–10] In the 2006 National Health Interview Survey, only 4% of U.S. adults had been told they had prediabetes.[8] Although 88 million U.S. adults 18 years or older had prediabetes in 2018, only 15.3% reported being told by a health professional that they had prediabetes.[9] Analysis of A1C data from the 2012 National Ambulatory Medical Care Survey that targeted adults aged >45 years without diagnosed diabetes (N = 11,167,004 weighted visits) showed a prediabetes prevalence of 33.6% by A1C criterion.[10] However, less than 1% of patients with A1C results in the prediabetes range had documentation of prediabetes status in their medical records.[10] Clearly, there is a great need for increased awareness of prediabetes screening among health professionals, particularly those engaged in primary care.

Once diagnosed, using fasting plasma glucose, an oral glucose tolerance test, or A1C values, the clinical significance of prediabetes needs to be communicated clearly to all affected individuals.[11] There is emerging evidence that awareness of prediabetes status may have salutary effects on health behavior and glucose tolerance, even without medical intervention.[12] During 5.5 years of follow-up (mean 2.62 years), 101 of 343 initially normoglycemic subjects who enrolled in the Pathobiology of Prediabetes in a Biracial Cohort (POP-ABC) study developed incident prediabetes and were notified, without any interventions. The remainder ($N = 242$) maintained normoglycemia during follow-up (control group). All participants were recalled after 18 months and, on retesting, significant differences were observed in interval changes in metabolic and behavioral data between the group who had received notification of incident prediabetes and the control group. Compared with the control group, the group with incident prediabetes had a lower fasting plasma glucose (−8.01 ± 1.11 vs. 2.02 ± 0.64 mg/dL, $P < 0.0001$), lower 2-h plasma glucose (−8.21 ± 3.34 vs. 8.53 ± 3.17 mg/dL, $P = 0.0004$), lower weight (−0.54 ± 0.72 vs. 2.77 ± 1.25 kg, $P = 0.006$), and lower waist circumference (−1.07 ± 0.78 vs. 1.78 ± 0.85 cm, $P = 0.001$).[12] The interval changes in fasting plasma glucose were significantly correlated with changes in weight and waist circumference ($r = 0.20$, $P = 0.01$). Analysis of food habits and physical activity data showed that the group notified of prediabetes status made significantly more changes toward healthier eating and increased activity during the interval between notification of prediabetes status and reevaluation.[12] Thus, passive communication of prediabetes status is associated with improvements in glucose and weight control, probably as a result of increased motivation to initiate self-directed lifestyle modification.[12] Once individuals have been diagnosed with prediabetes, appropriate referral for lifestyle counseling can follow, as recommended by the American Diabetes Association.[13,14]

Health care workers who become champions for diabetes prevention along with their primed families become conduits for the dissemination and diffusion of diabetes prevention ideas in targeted public spheres (hospital communities, established patients and their relatives, schools, neighborhoods, social media and outlets, religious forums, etc.). Because communities around the world have become familiar with the ravages of poorly controlled diabetes, it can be assumed that the public is preconditioned to be receptive to campaigns that promote the benefits of prevention and is motivated to avoid dreaded complications, such as blindness, amputation, kidney disease, and cardiovascular disease. Despite such a preconditioning of society regarding diabetes and its complications, the fact that type 2 diabetes can be prevented by modest lifestyle modification is yet to be widely recognized and promoted in communities around the world. That hiatus in the popular consciousness (in the face of the raging global epidemic of diabetes) presents an opportunity for leadership by health care professionals and civic leaders. Convincing and motivating large segments of society to take preventive action against diabetes requires coordinated efforts at the local, regional, state, national, and international leadership levels. A committed vision for a diabetes-free society promoted by ministries and departments of health, education, information, agriculture, finance, defense, and other governmental agencies could catalyze awareness and action at the population level. Collaboration from philanthropic and professional organizations and other nongovernmental bodies, especially local, national, and international diabetes associations, is critical for program building, facilitation, and scaling in the community. In that regard, the American Diabetes Association and the Centers for Disease Control and Prevention have led campaigns to increase public awareness about prediabetes.

Strategies for Diabetes Prevention in the Community

Seven key elements mostly distilled from the lifestyle intervention protocols of landmark diabetes prevention trials lend themselves to adaptation and translation in the community (Table 9.1). These keys to translation of diabetes prevention in the community are discussed in detail in the sections that follow.

Screening and selection of individuals at risk

Despite the raging global epidemic of diabetes, the majority of people do not currently have diabetes. Thus, applying a universal intervention strategy to the entire population would be inefficient, expensive, and wasteful of valuable resources. However, an approach targeted at individuals at high risk for developing type 2

Table 9.1—Translating Lifestyle Intervention for Diabetes Prevention in the Community

- Incorporate wellness and prevention education in school curriculum.
- Coordinate efforts at multiple levels within the society.
- Provide access to safe walking trails and well-kept, well-lit public parks.
- Increase nutritional education and food choices in neighborhoods.
- Enact policy changes that stimulate broad societal participation.
- Reward healthful behavior and discourage harmful behavior.
- Create community primary prevention or wellness centers.

Table 9.2—Risk Factors for Prediabetes and Type 2 Diabetes

- Family history of type 2 diabetes
- Overweight/obesity
- Sedentariness and physical inactivity
- Ethnicity
- History of gestational diabetes
- Delivery of baby weighing ≥9 lb
- High-normal fasting plasma glucose
- Hypertension
- Dyslipidemia
- Organ transplantation and immunosuppression
- Drug exposures: glucocorticoids, antipsychotics, HIV antiretroviral agents

diabetes would be more efficient. Such individuals are recognizable if they harbor one or more of the criteria that define prediabetes. The Da Qing study screened 110,660 men and women with oral glucose tolerance tests and enrolled 577 subjects with prediabetes (impaired glucose tolerance); the Diabetes Prevention Program screened more than 100,000 adults, using a four-step screening and recruitment process, to identify and enroll 3,243 eligible participants.[4,15] Thus, it is important to use a risk factor-based approach to identify individuals with prediabetes who may benefit from preventive intervention (Table 9.2). Family history of type 2 diabetes, overweight or obesity, and habitual physical inactivity are key clinical features that can be combined with blood glucose measurements to select at-risk individuals for diabetes prevention intervention. Indeed, all diabetes prevention trials targeted, screened, and enrolled such at-risk individuals, using well-known risk factors for type 2 diabetes. The merit of that approach was proven by the outcomes of those trials: participants randomized to placebo did in fact develop type 2 diabetes as predicted (10–12% per year in the Diabetes Prevention Program and ~18% per year in the Indian Diabetes Prevention Program-1).[3,6] Furthermore, studies that have applied the Diabetes Prevention Program approach in community settings have demonstrated the external validity of risk factor-based enrollment.[16,17]

Thus, the general criteria used for selecting at-risk individuals in the randomized controlled trials have proven to be of high fidelity and can be adopted for translation of diabetes prevention in the general populace. Specifically, a positive family history of type 2 diabetes in first-degree relatives, habitual sedentariness, overweight or obesity (using ethnic-specific BMI cutoffs), and a fasting plasma glucose in the range of 96–125 mg/dL would identify suitable individuals for enrollment in community diabetes prevention programs. The appropriate BMI cutoff for identifying overweight subjects is ethnic-specific: a BMI cutoff of >22 kg/m^2 is recommended for Asians, whereas a BMI cutoff of >25 kg/m^2 is appropriate for most other populations.[3] The age ranges targeted for inclusion in the published diabetes prevention trials were variable: >25 years for the Diabetes Prevention Program and Da Qing studies, 40–65 years for the Finnish study, and 30–55 years for the Indian trial.[3–5] Thus, none of the landmark diabetes prevention trials enrolled younger individuals with prediabetes. It is important to demonstrate efficacy of lifestyle intervention in preventing type 2 diabetes among children and adolescents with prediabetes, giving the increasing prevalence of type 2 diabetes in younger age-groups.[18,19] Until such pertinent studies are conducted, it is reasonable, on empirical grounds, for community diabetes prevention initiatives to lower the inclusive age for screening at-risk individuals well into the childhood and adolescent years. To control costs, the community efforts need to be coordinated with pediatric primary care providers. If any children and adolescents with prediabetes are identified through such screening programs, they should benefit from lifestyle intervention. A community family-based program[19] and a school-based program have demonstrated that obesity and diabetes risk factors can be decreased by lifestyle intervention in children and adolescents.[20] The school-based program was strictly not a diabetes prevention program, since the intervention was applied nonselectively to all sixth graders, instead of to a risk factor-based defined group. As a result, there was no change in blood glucose before and after the 3-year program; fasting glucose remained in the 93–94 mg/dL range throughout the program.[19] In the family-based program, lifestyle intervention was delivered to either mothers with a history of gestational diabetes or mothers and their adolescent children (aged 8–15 years).[19] The primary outcome was a change in weight at 3 months in adults; other outcomes included A1C, lipids, and blood pressure. Post-intervention assessments were made at 6 and 12 months. The children showed a reduction in BMI (−1.77, $P = 0.014$) that was sustained for 12 months post-intervention, but there was no weight change in the mothers. Significant reductions were observed in A1C levels in the mothers and their children, which were sustained for up to 1 year after intervention.[20]

As already noted in the report from the POP-ABC study, awareness of prediabetes status may induce self-directed beneficial changes in health behavior.[12] Those changes include healthier food choices and increased physical activity; the latter averaged a significant increase of 6 MET-hours per week in physical activity among POP-ABC participants who were informed of their prediabetes status.[12] In a national survey of U.S. adults who had been told that they had prediabetes, 68% reported active measures to control their weight, 55% reported becoming more physically active, 60% reported lower intake of fat, and 42% reported combined dietary and exercise changes.[8] In another report, also based on a U.S. national survey, data on A1C and fasting plasma glucose levels were checked against self-reported diabetes and prediabetes diagnosis to assess awareness status.[21] The investigators analyzed 24-h dietary recall data in relation to awareness of diabetes or prediabetes status. Compared with people with undiagnosed diabetes, individuals with diagnosed diabetes reported decreasing the intake of carbohydrates and increasing protein consumption.[21] However, the authors observed no significant differences in macronutrient intake between individuals with diagnosed or undiagnosed prediabetes and concluded that knowledge of glycemic status induced healthier dietary patterns for people with diabetes but not those with prediabetes.[21] Clearly, additional studies are needed to provide definitive answers. Nonetheless, it seems reasonable to expect that awareness of an incipient condition, such as prediabetes, could trigger healthier choices, at least in some individuals.

Despite the seemingly spontaneous beneficial changes that could be triggered by awareness of prediabetes status, sadly, most people with prediabetes are unaware of their condition.[8–10] The urgent need for greater awareness of prediabetes among health care workers and the general population cannot be overstated. Although the oral glucose tolerance test was the gold-standard screening method for the diabetes prevention trials, using a clinical profile, supported by any objective measure (fasting plasma glucose, oral glucose tolerance test, or A1C), is more pragmatic for identifying candidates for lifestyle modification in large-scale community operations.[14]

Delivery of physical activity intervention

The efficacious dose of physical activity in lifestyle intervention programs for diabetes prevention is characterized by moderate intensity (~55% Vo_2 max) and a duration of 150 min/week (~30 min daily in the Diabetes Prevention Program). The Diabetes Prevention Program exercise goal of 150 min/week was equal to that prescribed in the Da Qing studies but lower than the 210 min/week prescribed in the Finnish study.[3–5] Although 150 min/week is the recommended goal, significant metabolic benefits can be derived from shorter sessions of activity (e.g., 10–15 min spread across two or three periods during the day).[14,22] Communicating these benefits along with the impact of brief exercise on cognitive function[23] and longevity[24] is crucial when engaging sedentary individuals and is particularly valuable for advancing time-pressed individuals from the precontemplative stage toward readiness for change.[1,2,14,22–24]

Initially, Diabetes Prevention Program lifestyle participants were screened with submaximal cardiac stress tests before initiating a physical activity program.[3] However, such cardiac stress testing was not needed in other diabetes prevention trials, and the lifestyle modification programs have been well tolerated,[3–6] without untoward cardiovascular events or musculoskeletal injuries. A routine requirement for prescreening with cardiac stress before enrollment in a lifestyle-based

Table 9.3—Energy Expended in Various Physical Activities Expressed in METs per Hour

Activity	METs/h
Walking slowly (<2 mph)	2.0
Light gardening	2.0
General house cleaning	3.0
Walking briskly, 3 mph	3.3
Heavy yard work or gardening	4.0
Climbing stairs	4.0
Bicycling, casual, <10 mph	4.0
Dancing (ballet or modern)	4.8
Mowing the lawn with hand mower	6.0
Shoveling snow	6
Strenuous hiking	6–7
Rowing or kayaking	6–8
Skiing downhill	6–8
Bicycling, 10–16 mph	6–10
Aerobic calisthenics	6–10
Singles tennis	7–12
Swimming, crawl, slow	8.0
Running, 8 mph	13.5

MET is the ratio of the activity metabolic rate to the resting metabolic rate. One MET = 1 kcal/kg/h, which is equivalent to the energy spent sitting quietly.

diabetes prevention program would hamper any meaningful broad translation in the community. Walking was the preferred activity for most participants in these studies, but several other physical activities can improve aerobic fitness and glucoregulation (Table 9.3).

The motivation to partake in regular physical activity is often in competition with the demands of earning a livelihood. As rates of voluntary physical activity are remarkably low in urbanized communities,[25–28] creative strategies are needed to motivate exercise behavior and facilitate access to venues for safe physical activity. The randomized diabetes prevention clinical trials often used the expert services of nutritionists, dietitians, and exercise physiologists for delivery of the lifestyle intervention program. That is not feasible for large-scale community programs; therefore, lay individuals must be trained to deliver the dietary, physical activity, and other components of the lifestyle program. Globally, many communities lack the infrastructure for large-scale implementation of physical activity—well-maintained public parks, safe walkways, biking trails, health and fitness clubs, public swimming pools, or other places for physical activity. One innovative approach to the problem of space for physical activity is to consider partnerships with schools and houses of religious worship, so that their large real estate can be used for diabetes prevention activity after school hours and during nonworship days. Already, the personnel and physical space at YMCA locations in several communities across the United States are being deployed for diabetes prevention initiatives.[17]

Environmental challenges in some parts of the world can pose additional barriers to regular outdoor exercise. In addition, some cultures consider corpulence as reflecting high social status and freedom from wasting diseases (such as malnutrition, HIV/AIDS, and tuberculosis). In such settings, promoting efforts to lose weight may not be well received. There is also a less obvious socioeconomic angle that associates regular exercise with the privileged elite class. All these cultural (mis-)perceptions must be confronted with aggressive health education and public awareness campaigns. Such campaigns should emphasize the risks of obesity and promote the health benefits of modest increases in physical activity. The narrative must shift away from the notion of exercise as indulgent leisure of the bourgeoisie to one where exercise is embraced as an engine of wellness and health preservation and disease prevention among the proletariat. Civic and local government leaders should mobilize and model community resources for participatory health promotion and wellness. Whenever appropriate, participatory physical activity and health promotion should be built into scheduled cultural festivals and other activities. The latter could include student-teacher and parent-child low- to moderate-intensity sporting events, parades, pageants, mini-carnivals, and other civic celebrations.

The infatuation of the citizenry with certain national sporting events can be exploited for health promotion and diabetes prevention. The example of Brazil and soccer is worthy of emulation. Vieira de Sousa et al.[29] launched an innovative physical activity intervention among middle-aged patients with type 2 diabetes at the University of Sao Paulo, Brazil.[29] The program involved participation in 40-min soccer sessions 3 times per week for 12 weeks. The author was privileged to observe (and later join) the team sport during a tour as Visiting Professor at the University of Sao Paulo (Fig. 9.1). The enthusiasm among the group was infectious. It was a delight to witness middle-aged men and women running around in their bright soccer uniforms, trying to reenact the prowess of Pele, the legendary Brazilian soccer icon! Focused on scoring or defending goals, none of the patients consciously thought of the event as an exercise prescription. They were simply having fun. Post-study evaluation showed comprehensive improvements in cardiometabolic end points.[29] It is doubtful whether the same enthusiasm would have occurred had these patients been referred for routine exercise counseling. Interestingly, the physical activity component of the Malmö diabetes prevention study conducted among Swedish men also used a range of sporting activities that included

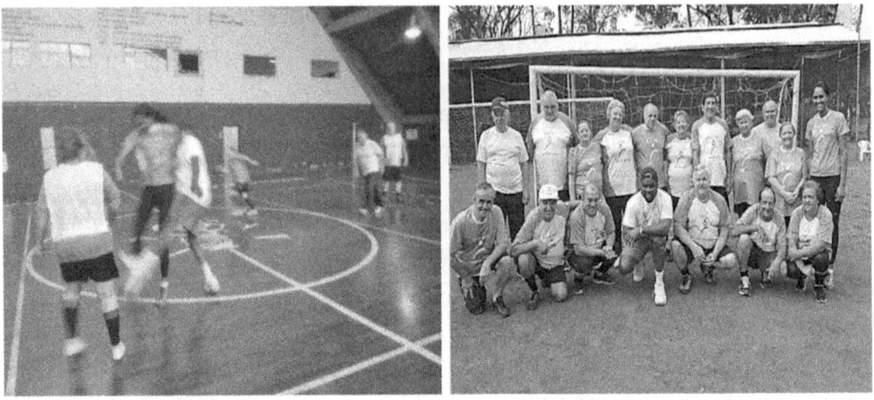

Figure 9.1—Modeling team sport as a vehicle for delivery of physical activity: the Brazilian soccer example, University of Sao Paulo, 2014.

calisthenics, soccer, and badminton.[30] Low- to medium-intensity activity programs designed around competitive team sports, such as soccer, basketball, volleyball, badminton, cricket, rugby, hockey, tennis, and other specific national sporting events could serve as popular vehicles for the large-scale translation of physical activity intervention for diabetes prevention in the community. Clearly, physicians, clinical researchers, and other health workers must get involved in prevention by creatively reimagining delivery methods for lifestyle intervention.

Frequent contacts

Face-to-face contact was the primary interaction mode between prediabetes subjects and lifestyle interventionists in the major diabetes prevention trials. The frequency of such contacts during the diabetes prevention programs varied from weekly, monthly, and bimonthly, to quarterly, depending on the specific study and phase of study. A significant positive correlation was reported between the frequency of attendance of scheduled face-to-face meetings and the magnitude of weight loss in behavioral studies.[31,32] In the Diabetes Prevention Program, the greatest weight loss occurred during the first 6 months when intensive lifestyle intervention participants were counseled face-to-face during weekly sessions.[3] After the frequency of visits was decreased to monthly sessions, weight regain occurred. However, participants in the Finnish Diabetes Prevention Study and the Da Qing study received lifestyle counseling every 2–3 months yet achieved diabetes risk reduction outcomes that were similar or close to the 58% reduction observed in the Diabetes Prevention Program.[3,5] It seems that face-to-face contact at some frequency is desirable for successful translation of diabetes prevention intervention. The mechanisms for the contribution of such contacts to the success of diabetes prevention programs could include the development of "bonding" through favorable dynamics between lifestyle coaches and participants. Also, the expectation of being weighed and measured could motivate adherence to recommended diet and exercise among participants. The optimal frequency of physical contacts necessary for successful diabetes prevention in the community remains to be determined and could well be different across regions of the world because of socioeconomic, cultural, or religious factors. Ideally, local data would need to be generated in pilot studies in different communities, to inform the selection of best or optimal practices.

Clearly, a requirement of frequent face-to-face counseling would hamper large-scale translation of diabetes prevention practices for the hundreds of millions of adults with prediabetes globally. Mixed or hybrid lifestyle intervention delivery methods that combine low-frequency physical contacts with remote contacts is conceivable as a cost-saving and convenient option. Community diabetes prevention initiatives that involve fewer face-to-face sessions in group format, supplemented by virtual contacts (SMS text messaging, e-mail, social media, or web-based platforms), could be less expensive to run, more convenient for participants, and more scalable. Emerging data from Australia, the United States, Europe, and Asia indicate that web-based lifestyle modification programs have modest but variable effects on weight loss.[33–41] In general, the web-based or virtual weight loss programs involve an initial introductory face-to-face session during which participants receive training on Internet navigation and login procedures along with written instructions. Each participant receives a unique password-protected access and identification code to the program website. Issues pertaining to web security and the risk of potential breaches in confidentiality of data uploaded to the program website are also discussed during the introductory session. Participants may also receive a one-time face-to-face lifestyle counseling session on standard behavioral weight-control instruction on diet, exercise, and behavior change during the introductory meeting.

In a basic Internet program, the website provides a primer or tutorial on weight loss strategies (in written or video format) along with helpful tips and resources, including meal plans, sample menus, and tools for tracking weight, calories, and exercise activity. The website also provides links to additional pertinent information on weight management.[33–41] The tutorials and links are updated regularly with new information, and participants are prompted by e-mail to upload their weight to the website at regular intervals (usually weekly). Each participant receives regular feedback on progress with weight loss.[33–41] The basic Internet program can be supplemented with behavioral e-counseling.[33–41] The latter involves more frequent (daily to weekly) self-monitoring and reporting of additional data by participants (such as calorie intake, nature and duration of exercise, challenges and barriers, etc.) and regular feedback from a counselor.[33] The e-mail feedback from the counselor focuses on the participant's self-monitoring dietary and activity record and is geared toward providing decision support, suggestions for change, or ideas on how to overcome barriers. Objective monitoring of adiposity and biochemical end points (including weight, waist circumference, or blood glucose) usually occurs during assessment visits to the clinic at scheduled intervals.[33–41]

Comparing a web-based intervention to face-to-face counseling sessions, some studies have observed similar efficacy in maintaining weight loss, but other workers have reported less impressive weight loss outcome with Internet intervention compared to physical contacts.[33–42] Wing et al.[36] compared the effect of Internet delivery versus face-to-face intervention on the pattern of weight regain in people who had lost ~20 kg within the 2 years preceding initiation of the study. In all, 314 such participants were assigned randomly to one of three groups: a control group, a face-to-face intervention group, and an Internet-based intervention group. The control group received quarterly newsletters on healthy habits by mail. Other than mode of delivery, the behavioral management content of the programs in the two intervention groups was identical, as was the frequency of contact between counsellors and participants in each group. Participants were then followed for 18 months, with the primary outcome being change in weight. The investigators found that the mean weight regained was lowest in the face-to-face group (2.5 ± 6.7 kg) compared with the Internet group (4.7 ± 8.6 kg) and the control group (4.9 ± 6.5 kg).[36] However, the proportion of subjects who regained ≥2.3 kg during the 18-month follow-up period was significantly lower in the Internet (54.8%; absolute difference 18%, 95% CI 5–30%, $P = 0.008$) and face-to-face (45.7%; absolute difference 27%, 95% CI 14–39%, $P < 0.001$) groups compared with the control group (72.4%). Thus, an Internet-based intervention did not match the efficacy of face-to-face intervention, although it was superior to control in attenuating the magnitude of recrudescence in weight.

Harvey-Berino et al.[35] investigated the effectiveness of a weight maintenance program conducted over the Internet in 122 overweight adults (age 48.4 ± 9.6, BMI 32.2 ± 4.5 kg/m^2). All participants received a 6-month in-person lifestyle management program and then were assigned randomly to receive one of three options for maintenance support for 12 months: in-person support at minimal frequency of visits, in-person support at high frequency of visits, or support over the Internet. The randomization to maintenance support options occurred before commencement of the initial 6-month in-person intervention that all participants underwent. Minimal frequency in-person support consisted of monthly 1-h in-person sessions with the lifestyle therapist the first 6 months only of the 12-month weight maintenance condition. The in-person support at high frequency consisted of biweekly sessions with the lifestyle therapist throughout the 12-month maintenance period. The Internet support group uploaded self-monitoring data to the study website, viewed an instructional video, and met every 2 weeks for a group chat, facilitated by the group therapist. Between group chat sessions, the group therapist maintained e-mail communication with participants in the Internet support group to obtain weekly self-monitoring data and to provide general support. The investigators reported that weight loss at the end of the initial 6 months of in-person treatment did not differ significantly by assigned maintenance group.[35] After the in-person weight management, participants in all three groups experienced weight regain during the initial 6 months of the maintenance period. The investigators observed that the amount of weight regained during that 6-month period was significantly greater among subjects in the Internet support group (2.2 ± 3.8 kg) compared with the frequent in-person support group (0.0 ± 4.0 kg). The participants were then followed up under the three different weight loss support strategies for additional 6 months, making a total of 12 months of observation after the initial 6 months of in-person sessions. The overall weight loss from baseline at the end of the 12-month maintenance period was significantly lower in the Internet support group (−5.7 ± 5.9 kg) compared with the minimal in-person support group (−10.4 ± 9.3 kg) and the frequent in-person support group (−10.4 ± 6.3 kg).[35] The investigators concluded that Internet support was less effective at promoting long-term maintenance of weight loss than minimal or frequent in-person support by a lifestyle counselor.[35] The authors noted that attendance of scheduled counseling sessions during the 12-month maintenance period was lower in the Internet group than the frequent in-person support group (39 vs. 54%, $P = 0.04$), which could have affected the results.

In people with diagnosed type 2 diabetes, a meta-analysis of web-based interventions on dietary behavior change and glycemic control showed a modest aggregate benefit of web-based interventions compared with usual care.[38] Five studies (enrolling a total of 1,056 adults with type 2 diabetes) were included in the meta-analysis.[38] Of the latter, four studies reported significant improvements in dietary behavior (healthier food choices and reductions in carbohydrates, saturated fat, and overall fat intake), and three studies reported significant decreases in weight ranging from −2.3 to −12.7 kg as well as A1C ranging from −0.3% to −0.8%.[38] Thus, although the studies included were few, the overall trend favored benefits from web-based interventions regarding body weight and glycemic control in people with type 2 diabetes.[38] Given that asymptomatic individuals with prediabetes may be differently motivated than people with diabetes, it is unclear whether the conclusions from the meta-analysis can be extrapolated to those with prediabetes. However, meta-analyses of web-based behavioral interventions that enrolled overweight or obese subjects without diabetes do provide support for the overall benefit of virtual weight management, although there was heterogeneity in the effectiveness of web-based interventions across different studies.[39,40]

In a meta-analysis that included 23 studies (total enrollment of 8,697 overweight or obese participants), content delivery via the Internet was associated with a modest but significant additional weight loss compared with non-web user control groups (−0.68 kg, $P = 0.03$).[40] However, stratified analysis showed that the effectiveness of web-based intervention was most evident when that mode was used as an adjunct to standard obesity care (additional aggregate weight change of −1.00 kg in the Internet group).[40] In contrast, when web-based intervention was used as a substitute for standard face-to-face lifestyle counseling, the weight trajectory was not beneficial (additional aggregate weight change of +1.27 kg in the Internet group).[40] In general, greater attendance and use of website features appear to predict greater weight loss; however, the pooled meta-analysis data also suggest that the effectiveness of web-based intervention on weight loss tends to diminish after ~12 months of participation.[39,40]

A recent study compared the effectiveness of usual care versus either an online weight management program or a combined online weight management program plus in-person support by trained lay community workers (population health management).[41] Participants in the usual care group received general information about weight management by mail, and those in the online weight management group received a web-based behavioral intervention program. The third group received combined web-based intervention and weight-focused population health management. The latter comprised additional motivation and support from nonclinical lay community workers.[41] Using cluster randomization, the investigators enrolled 840 participants from 15 primary care practices in the United States The mean age of the cohort was 59.3 ± 8.6 years, with a BMI range of 27 to <40 kg/m^2; most participants were female (60%) or white (76.8%). The primary outcome was a change in body weight at 12 months of follow-up. The results showed that the mean weight change was −1.2 kg (95% CI −2.1 to −0.3 kg) in the usual care group, −1.9 kg (95% CI −2.6 to −1.1 kg) in the online intervention-only group, and −3.1 kg (95% CI −3.7 to −2.5 kg) in the combined online and population health management intervention group. These changes were significantly different by treatment groups ($P < 0.001$). The percentage of participants who had a weight loss of 5% or greater was 14.9% (95% CI 10.2–19.6%) in the usual care group, 20.8% (95% CI 14.5–27.2%) in the online program only group, and 32.3% (95% CI 25.8–38.8%) in the combined intervention, again significantly different by treatment groups.[41]

Thus, a mixed or hybrid model involving Internet delivery of lifestyle intervention supplemented with some form of in-person support seems appealing, although further evaluation is required to determine the best option for delivering diabetes prevention through lifestyle intervention in the community. There is also the vexing issue of "digital divide" that precludes numerous individuals from disadvantaged communities from participating in web-based initiatives. Based on the variable reports on the efficacy of web-based lifestyle intervention programs and related socioeconomic barriers, some level of face-to-face counseling would need to be built in to the format for lifestyle intervention for diabetes prevention in the community. Pending the availability of evidence-based data, a mixed model of in-person counseling sessions, supplemented with remote delivery methods, can be tested and adopted, if proven to be effective.

Delivery of dietary intervention

In general, the dietary approach to preventing type 2 diabetes focused on reducing total calories (by 500–700 kcal/day) and total and saturated fat and increasing intake of dietary fiber. Substantial dietary education was delivered to participants, to help them understand food labels and use the information on macronutrient composition to maintain a healthy eating pattern.[3] Written material containing information on caloric content of common foods was provided to participants. Such information is now widely available as teaching tools and can be accessed by people with prediabetes or clinicians interested in steering such individuals toward healthier eating patterns. Examples include the American Diabetes Association's Diabetes Food Hub (https://www.diabetesfoodhub.org), *The Diabetes Carbohydrate & Fat Gram Guide* (ISBN 9781580405553), and the Centers for Disease Control and Prevention's National Diabetes Prevention Program (https://www.cdc.gov/diabetes/prevention/index.html). Dietary counseling was typically delivered during face-to-face visits, individually or in groups. As discussed in the previous section, there is a documented correlation between frequency of counseling visits and the magnitude of weight loss in behavioral studies,[31,32] although the optimal frequency of such visits remains to be determined. It is reassuring that the Finnish Diabetes Prevention Study that used quarterly lifestyle counseling sessions achieved exactly similar results (58% reduction in type 2 diabetes risk) as another study that involved more frequent visits.[3,5] Thus, after initiation of the dietary intervention, maintenance visits at approximately 3-month intervals may be sufficient to yield desirable results in a community setting. Depending on available resources, the frequency of face-to-face visits could even be less, if the program is supplemented with remote contacts. There is evidence that web-based lifestyle modification programs may be beneficial for weight loss maintenance, although the reports have been somewhat discordant.[33–42]

There are some challenges besetting dietary intervention for diabetes prevention in developing countries, where the burden of future diabetes is predicted to be greatest. Many low- and middle-income regions of the world do not have adequate strengths in trained personnel (physicians, physician assistants, nurses, culturally adapted dietitians and medical nutritionists, exercise physiologists, etc.) to staff community diabetes prevention initiatives. Such countries may also lack the practice of mandatory food labeling (the result of legislation passed decades ago in Western countries), and nutritional information may be lacking for many local staple foods. Even where food labeling exists, the likelihood of comprehending and applying the information to drive healthy eating patterns may be negated by low rates of general and health literacy. Furthermore, most residents of rural and even urban areas patronize informal retail markets that sell staples (especially grains, flour, corn, cereal, rice, beans, cassava powder [gari], and other tuber-derived staples) that do not even offer standardized packaging.

The long-term solution to the challenges requires good governance and efficient national planning. For the immediate and foreseeable future, the approach to overcoming these impediments to dietary lifestyle intervention calls for creative thinking, rather than almost futile transplantation of a Diabetes Prevention Program–type intervention to the developing world. Effective dietary intervention strategies for diabetes prevention in developing countries must anticipate and overcome or circumvent the aforementioned translational obstacles. Much is needed by way of locally generated pilot and feasibility research into acceptable and successful forms of dietary modification. For instance, the use of a visual (pictorial) approach to dietary modification, instead of text-based format, may overcome the barrier of low literacy in some communities.

The plate method[43] popularized by the U.S. Department of Agriculture can be evaluated and adapted to local dietary norms as the basis for teaching portion control.[44] The Dietary Guidelines for Americans, issued by the U.S. Department of Agriculture, advocates a simple plate method, with half of the plate to be filled with fruits and vegetables; the other half is divided roughly equally between grains and protein[44] (Fig. 9.2). The plate method is an attractive visual model for teaching portion control and healthy eating dietary habits and could be particularly effective in low-literacy communities.

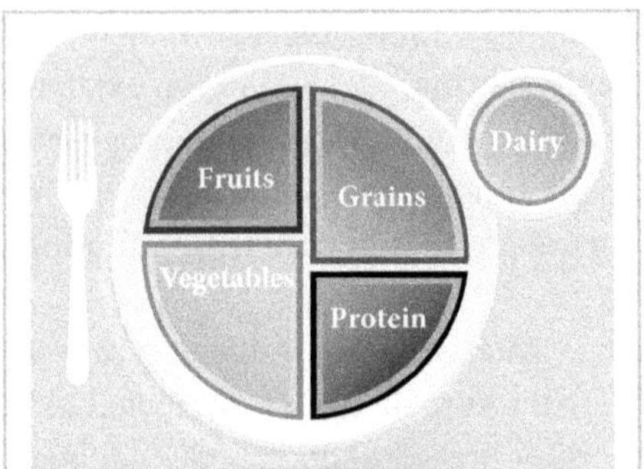

Fruits: Any fruit or 100% fruit juice counts as part of the fruit group. Fruits may be fresh, canned, frozen, or dried and may be whole, cut-up, or pureed. The amount of fruit you need to eat depends on age, sex, and level of physical activity. The amount each person needs can vary between 1 and 2 cups each day, and higher for very physically active people.
Vegetables: Any vegetable or 100% vegetable juice counts as a member of the vegetable group. Vegetables may be raw or cooked; fresh, frozen, canned, or dried/dehydrated; and may be whole, cut-up, or mashed. Based on their nutrient content, vegetables are organized into five subgroups: dark-green vegetables, starchy vegetables, red and orange vegetables, beans and peas, and other vegetables. The amount of vegetables needed can vary between 1 and 3 cups daily.
Grains: Any food made from wheat, rice, oats, cornmeal, barley, or another cereal grain is a grain product. Bread, pasta, oatmeal, breakfast cereals, tortillas, and grits are examples of grain products. Grains are divided into whole grains and refined grains. Whole grains contain the entire grain kernel — the bran, germ, and endosperm (e.g., whole-wheat flour, oatmeal, brown rice). Refined grains (e.g., white flour, white bread, white rice) have been milled to improve shelf-life, a process that removes the bran and germ as well as dietary fiber, iron, and many B vitamins. Most refined grains are reinforced with B vitamins and iron after processing, but fiber is not added back. The amount of grains needed can vary between 3- and 8-oz equivalents, at least half of which should be whole grains.
Protein: Meat, poultry, seafood, beans and peas, eggs, processed soy products, nuts, and seeds are considered part of the protein group. Note that beans and peas are also part of the vegetable group. The recommended protein intake for healthy people can vary between 2- and 6.5-oz equivalents each day and higher for very physically active people.
Dairy: All fluid milk products, milk derivatives (such as yogurt and cheese), and calcium-fortified soy milk are part of the dairy group. Foods made from milk that have little to no calcium, such as cream cheese, cream, and butter, are not part of the Dairy Group. The amount of dairy intake depends on age, and varies between 2 and 3 cups each day.

Figure 9.2—The plate method of healthy eating. For more information on recommended daily intake, examples of fruits, vegetables, grains, protein, and dairy, and to access an interactive healthy eating app, please visit www.choosemyplate.gov.

Mediterranean diet and intermittent fasting

Dietary practices that were not specifically tested in the landmark diabetes prevention trials, such as intermittent fasting and adoption of the Mediterranean diet, may nonetheless be worthy of consideration in the overall lifestyle modification strategy. The Mediterranean-style eating pattern (based on vegetables, fruits, nuts, seeds, legumes, whole grains, herbs, seafood, and extra virgin olive oil) has been associated with beneficial effects on weight control and cardiometabolic end points. In studies among overweight/obese subjects, the Mediterranean-style diet has consistently resulted in greater weight loss than general lifestyle counseling. In one study that enrolled 120 obese women and followed them for 2 years, participants who received education on Mediterranean-style diet and exercise showed greater weight loss than a control group who received general information about healthy food and exercise (14 vs. 3 kg, $P < 0.001$).[45] In other trials, participants randomized to a Mediterranean diet supplemented with extra-virgin olive oil experienced ~40% reduction in the incidence of type 2 diabetes compared with participants assigned to a low-fat control diet.[46–48] Thus, a Mediterranean-style eating pattern can be included in the dietary intervention curriculum for diabetes prevention in the community. The expanded flexibility of dietary options is likely to attract a broader base of interested candidates willing to participate in lifestyle modification.

Intermittent fasting is another dietary intervention approach that was not tested in the standard diabetes prevention trials. Intermittent fasting has a long history rooted in human cultural and religious traditions.[49–52] In modern times, intermittent fasting has been evaluated as a means of improving weight control and clinical outcomes.[53–58] Although definitions vary somewhat, intermittent fasting generally refers to a practice where individuals fast for 24 h every other day or for 16 h daily. Under this plan, the last meal of the day is eaten at 8:00 P.M. and fasting is maintained until noon the next day. The feeding commences from noon and ends at 8:00 P.M. Water and zero-calorie beverages are allowed during the fasting hours, but there are no specific restrictions during feeding hours. Specific studies of the effects of intermittent fasting in people with prediabetes are scant, but a recent systematic review suggests that intermittent fasting can be an effective adjunct for weight loss and glucose control in patients with type 2 diabetes.[59] There is evidence that restricting feeding times and extending interprandial intervals can promote weight loss via modulation of the gut microbiome.[60] Calorie restriction also serves as a potent activator of sirtuin, a gene involved in the regulation of energy metabolism and longevity.[61]

Self-monitoring

As part of the research protocol, participants in diabetes prevention trials maintained daily records of their intake of meals and snacks and minutes spent performing various physical activities each day.[3] Those records were reviewed by research staff during study visits, and appropriate feedback was given to participants. Although paper records were used in the diabetes prevention trials, digital tracking tools have since become available. Smartphone apps, such as MyFitnessPal, can now help track dietary intake and physical activity (www.myfitnesspal.com). Self-monitoring has been associated with successful long-term maintenance of weight loss.[62,63] In some studies, self-monitoring of blood glucose has also been linked to improved glycemic control.[64,65] Given the association between self-monitoring behavior and outcome, the regular detailed recording of food intake and exercise minutes could well have been one of the mediators of the excellent results obtained in the Diabetes Prevention Program and other diabetes prevention trials. The exact mechanisms linking the practice of self-monitoring to good outcome are unclear. It is plausible that adherence to self-monitoring reflects similar adherence behavior to the recommended diet and exercise regimens. Moreover, self-monitoring demonstrates close personal involvement in one's health, which indicates internality of locus of control, a harbinger of self-efficacy.[66,67] Finally, the feedback from the review of self-monitored data can have a powerful heuristic effect in guiding food choices and lifestyle decisions.

Could there be a possible downside to self-monitoring? For most people in psychic equilibrium, there should not be any stress from frequent self-monitoring of nutrient intake and physical activity. Given its role as a component of diabetes prevention protocols, it is prudent to incorporate self-monitoring in a community-based diabetes prevention campaign. Detailed accounting of the types, portions (serving sizes), and frequency of foods and snacks consumed and time spent on various physical activities should be the goal of self-monitoring. The use of home scales for regular self-weighing should be encouraged, and such data should be included in monitoring logs as well. In people with low literacy, family members, friends, and neighbors can be mobilized to help with record entry. Pictorial methods can be developed for capturing dietary and exercise data. The now globally ubiquitous cell phone can also be deployed as a recording and transmission device for self-monitored data via SMS text messages. Of course, as already stated, mobile phone apps are now available to support self-monitoring. Of importance, self-monitoring is effective in producing desired results only when the results are used to trigger behavior change. Thus, regular review of self-monitored data and appropriate feedback by clinicians and lifestyle interventionists is a crucial component of the process.

Weight loss goal-setting

The weight loss goal for lifestyle participants in the Diabetes Prevention Program and Finnish Diabetes Prevention Study was a 5–7% decrease in weight at enrollment.[3,5] The 7% weight loss target was achieved within 6 months of initiation of Diabetes Prevention Program lifestyle intervention but was not sustained. At the end of ~3 years of follow-up, the mean weight loss was ~4%.[3] In further analysis, the Diabetes Prevention Program investigators explored the contribution of changes in weight, diet, and physical activity on the risk of progression from prediabetes to type 2 diabetes among the participants assigned to intensive lifestyle intervention (N = 1,079; mean age 50.6 years, BMI 33.9 kg/m^2).[68] The findings showed that weight loss was the dominant predictor of decreased type 2 diabetes hazard among intensive lifestyle participants. The hazard ratio associated with each 5-kg weight loss was 0.42 (95% CI 0.35–0.51, $P < 0.0001$). After adjusting for changes in diet and physical activity, each 1-kg weight loss predicted a 16% reduction in diabetes risk.[68] Congruently, the magnitude of weight loss was positively correlated with decreased consumption of fat and increased physical activity. Furthermore, increased physical activity was an important mechanism for sustaining weight loss and preventing regain. Notably, among 495 participants who did not meet the weight loss target at year 1, the subgroup who achieved the physical activity target of ≥150 min/week experienced a 44% decrease in diabetes incidence.[68]

Taken together, these data underscore the rationale for targeting weight loss as a primary strategy for diabetes prevention in overweight or obese individuals with prediabetes. Increased physical activity is an important adjunct for maintaining weight loss; high levels of activity can also contribute to diabetes prevention, despite suboptimal weight loss. Unlike the Diabetes Prevention Program, participants in the Da Qing study and the Indian Diabetes Prevention Program-1 were enrolled with a relatively low baseline BMI (~23 kg/m^2) and did not lose an appreciable amount of weight during the years of lifestyle intervention. Despite the lack of evidence of weight loss, the Da Qing study and the Indian Diabetes Prevention Program-1 showed significant reductions in progression from prediabetes to type 2 diabetes with lifestyle intervention.[3,4,6] Additionally, the Da Qing study has reported impressive long-term data showing reductions in the incidence of microvascular and macrovascular complications and deaths associated with prior lifestyle intervention.[7] Thus, it is possible that even without demonstrable weight loss, participants receiving lifestyle intervention could have had unfavorable visceral body fat distribution at baseline that was ameliorated by the intervention. Furthermore, increased physical activity improves cardiorespiratory fitness, which is associated with improved cardiovascular outcomes and longevity. The improved cardiorespiratory fitness from moderate-intensity exercise can be observed 10 years after cessation of the intervention.[69,70] Based on these findings, community diabetes prevention programs should adopt a flexible approach that targets weight loss in overweight and obese people and weight maintenance in others, through optimization of diet and increased physical activity.

Smoking cessation

Cigarette smoking is associated with insulin resistance, increased cardiovascular disease, and increased risk of incident type 2 diabetes during longitudinal follow-up.[71–74] The hazard ratio for incident type 2 diabetes during 9 years of follow-up was 1.42 (95% CI 1.20–1.67) in the highest tertile of pack-years compared with never-smokers.[75] However, smoking cessation is associated with an increased risk of incident type 2 diabetes that peaks during the first 3 years and decreases to 0 at 12 years.[75–77] The transient increase in diabetes risk is attributable to weight gain in ex-smokers.[75–77] Cigarette smoking increases the risk of cardiovascular disease death up to four-fold among people with diabetes, depending on the amount smoked.[71] Poorer glycemic control and dyslipidemia also have been associated with smoking in patients with diabetes.[72,73] The dysmetabolic effects of cigarette smoking precede the development of diabetes; in fact, smoking has been identified as a risk factor for the metabolic syndrome.[74] Several mechanisms have been demonstrated or proposed to explain the association between smoking and increased risks of diabetes and cardiovascular disease. The list included induction of insulin resistance, increased hepatic lipase activity, suppression of protective HDL cholesterol levels, and chronic stress response. Other mechanisms include endothelial dysfunction and the vasoconstrictive effect of nicotine.[71–74] Thus, smoking cessation can be expected to ameliorate the noxious effects of nicotine and decrease cardiometabolic risk. People with prediabetes should be evaluated for tobacco use, and users should be encouraged to stop. Formal referral for tobacco cessation should be considered as part of the comprehensive management of prediabetes. Given the reported increase in diabetes risk during the first 3 years of smoking cessation, close monitoring and proactive intensification of lifestyle intervention is warranted in recent ex-smokers.[14] Additionally, evaluation and management of anxiety, depression, stress, and sleep impairment are advisable.

Community Diabetes Prevention Centers

Aspects of the key lifestyle modification that proved remarkably effective in delaying or preventing progression from prediabetes to type 2 diabetes, and sometimes even reversing prediabetes and restoring normal glucose regulation, in trials conducted in high-risk populations in China, India, Europe, the United States, New Zealand, and other countries are likely to be applicable to other regions of the world (including Africa, Latin America, Australia, New Zealand, the Middle East, and the Caribbean), where no randomized controlled diabetes prevention trials have yet been reported. However, some would argue that randomized controlled trials or pragmatic studies are needed in those latter countries, to inform best practices. Such studies, if feasible in those regions, would be informative and valuable. Nonetheless, given the strength of the evidence, there is little doubt that lifestyle modification focusing on healthy eating, increased physical activity, and weight loss (in individuals who are overweight or obese) would be beneficial in individuals with prediabetes in any region of the world. There is no evidence of racial/ethnic resistance to the efficacy of lifestyle intervention on diabetes prevention. In the Diabetes Prevention Program, the magnitude of diabetes risk reduction was similar among European Americans, African Americans, Hispanic Americans, Asian Americans, and Native American Indians.[3] Thus, the important question is, how can diabetes prevention be translated and organized in communities around the world?

Recall that the landmark diabetes prevention studies were designed as randomized controlled trials and conducted predominantly at tertiary academic medical centers. The study protocols required frequent clinic visits, and the study staff was comprised of highly trained experts, including physicians, nurses, dietitians, psychologists, exercise physiologists, and others. The studies needed substantial resources and support from institutions and funding agencies, and services were provided free of charge to participants. Many of these features would not be easily reproducible in the community. As such, structural adaptations (including use of laypersons to deliver interventions) would be needed for translating diabetes prevention in the community. The National Diabetes Prevention Program launched by the U.S. Centers for Disease Control and Prevention is a notable example. The Centers for Disease Control and Prevention has been training and certifying laypersons in the community to serve as lifestyle coaches for diabetes prevention.[78] Programs using trained laypersons to deliver adaptations of the Diabetes Prevention Program lifestyle intervention to groups (rather than one-on-one sessions) in the community have shown promising results.[16,17,19]

The current and projected future global burdens of diabetes and prediabetes call for a broad and vigorous response at the community level, particularly in developing countries that would be disproportionately saddled with a future diabetes burden. Organizing such a broad and vigorous response to the diabetes pandemic around Community Diabetes Prevention Centers (CDPCs) seems efficient.[79] The establishment of CDPCs at several locations in sub-Saharan Africa, the Middle East and North Africa, the Caribbean, India and South Asia, the Pacific Rim, South and Central America, Australia and New Zealand, and in communities inhabited by high-risk populations in Europe and North America would reflect the needed broad and vigorous response. CDPCs can serve as focal points for the dispensation of educational initiatives and dissemination of diabetes prevention practices. Operationally, the CDPCs can be administered and staffed by the noncommunicable diseases branch of ministries and departments of health, or through partnerships with nongovernmental voluntary agencies and local diabetes associations. The primary purpose of CDPCs would be to facilitate the creation and implementation of culturally and regionally appropriate models of the delivery of diabetes prevention at the grassroots level. Referral to CDPCs by primary care providers can be based on a risk factor approach that focuses on family history of diabetes and the other well-known risk markers. Individuals with diagnosed type 2 diabetes, who have experienced the condition first-hand, can be motivated to serve as conduits for referral of family members to CDPCs for prediabetes screening and intervention.

Who will pay for diabetes prevention services?

Costs analysis by the Diabetes Prevention Program investigators confirmed that preventing type 2 diabetes was cost-effective for society.[80–83] Over 3 years of intervention, the direct medical costs associated with the Diabetes Prevention Program were $79 per subject (placebo arm), $2,542 per subject (metformin arm), and $2,780 in the lifestyle group.[80] Analysis of Diabetes Prevention Program costs over a longer term showed that lifestyle intervention remained cost-effective and metformin was potentially cost-saving.[81] Cost analysis in the Indian Diabetes Prevention Program also showed that lifestyle intervention was cost-effective: the reported total cost of identifying one person with prediabetes (impaired glucose tolerance) was $117, and the direct medical costs were $61 per person (control arm) and $225 (lifestyle intervention arm).[82] The cost of preventing one case of type 2 diabetes through lifestyle modification in India was $1,052.[82]

Of note, the Diabetes Prevention Program, the Indian Diabetes Prevention Program, and other randomized controlled trials were resource intensive. Strategies for lowering the costs associated with diabetes prevention in communities around the world include delivery of lifestyle intervention to groups and use of trained laypersons instead of health professionals. In addition, rationalization of contact frequency, supplementation of in-person contacts with remote electronic substitutes, and use of unoccupied community spaces (after-hours school premises, or churches and religious premises on nonworship days), among other creative initiatives, could decrease costs. Furthermore, health care systems based on government or commercial insurance coverage could explore issuing subsidies and discounts to stimulate healthy habits, including enrollment in diabetes prevention programs for individuals with prediabetes. Sadly, even with a drastically scaled-down costs model, pervasive poverty and competition from other national priorities could militate against the highly desirable establishment of diabetes prevention initiatives. Given this reality, the impetus falls on partnerships among leaders from the private sector, nongovernmental agencies, local and international charitable organizations, industry, and other entities to save humanity from the scourge of diabetes by promoting and supporting diabetes prevention initiatives in resource-poor countries.

References

1. Prochaska JO, Velicer WF. The transtheoretical model of health behavior change. *Am J Health Promot* 1997;12:38–48
2. Velicer WF, Brick LA, Fava JL, Prochaska JO. Testing 40 predictions from the transtheoretical model again, with confidence. *Multivariate Behav Res* 2013;48:220–240
3. Knowler WC, Barrett-Connor E, Fowler SE, et al.; Diabetes Prevention Program Research Group. Reduction in the incidence of type 2 diabetes with lifestyle intervention or metformin. *N Engl J Med* 2002;346:393–403
4. Pan XR, Li GW, Hu YH, et al. Effects of diet and exercise in preventing NIDDM in people with impaired glucose tolerance: the Da Qing IGT and Diabetes Study. *Diabetes Care* 1997;20:537–544
5. Tuomilehto J, Lindström J, Eriksson JG, et al. Prevention of type 2 diabetes mellitus by changes in lifestyle among subjects with impaired glucose tolerance. *N Engl J Med* 2001;344:1343–1350
6. Ramachandran A, Snehalatha C, Mary S, et al. The Indian Diabetes Prevention Program shows that lifestyle modification and metformin prevent type 2 diabetes in Asian Indian subjects with impaired glucose tolerance (IDPP-1). *Diabetologia* 2006;49:289–297
7. Gong Q, Zhang P, Wang J, et al.; DaQing Diabetes Prevention Study Group. Morbidity and mortality after lifestyle intervention for people with impaired glucose tolerance: 30 year results of the Da Qing Diabetes Prevention Outcome Study. *Lancet Diabetes Endocrinol* 2019;7:45–461
8. Centers for Disease Control and Prevention. Self-reported prediabetes and risk-reduction activities: United States, 2006. *MMWR* 2008;57: 1203–1205
9. Centers for Disease Control and Prevention. *National Diabetes Statistics Report, 2020. Estimates of Diabetes and Its Burden in the United States.* Atlanta, GA, Centers for Disease Control and Prevention, U.S. Department of Health and Human Services. Available from https://www.cdc.gov/diabetes/pdfs/data/statistics/national-diabetes-statistics-report.pdf. Accessed 28 October 2020
10. Mainous AG, Tanner RJ, Baker R. Prediabetes diagnosis and treatment in primary care. *J Am Board Fam Med* 2016;29:283–285
11. Brannick B, Wynn A, Dagogo-Jack S. Prediabetes as a toxic environment for the initiation of microvascular and macrovascular complications. *Exp Biol Med (Maywood)* 2016;241:1323–1331
12. Owei I, Umekwe U, Ceesay F, Dagogo-Jack S. Awareness of prediabetes status and subsequent health behavior, body weight, and blood glucose levels. *J Am Board Fam Med* 2019;32:20–27

13. Nathan DM, Davidson MB, DeFronzo RA, et al. Impaired fasting glucose and impaired glucose tolerance. *Diabetes Care* 2007;30:753–759
14. American Diabetes Association. 3. Prevention or delay of type 2 diabetes: *Standards of Medical Care in Diabetes—2020. Diabetes Care* 2020;43: S32–S36
15. Rubin RR, Fujimoto WY, Marrero DG, et al.; DPP Research Group. The Diabetes Prevention Program: recruitment methods and results. *Control Clin Trials* 2002;23:157–171
16. Hays LM, Finch EA, Saha C, et al. Effect of self-efficacy on weight loss: a psychosocial analysis of a community-based adaptation of the diabetes prevention program lifestyle intervention. *Diabetes Spectr* 2014;27: 270–275
17. Finch EA, Kelly MS, Marrero DG, Ackermann RT. Training YMCA wellness instructors to deliver an adapted version of the Diabetes Prevention Program lifestyle intervention. *Diabetes Educ* 2009;35:224–228, 232
18. Kaufman FR. Type 2 diabetes mellitus in children and youth: a new epidemic. *J Pediatr Endocrinol Metab* 2002;15(Suppl. 2):737–744
19. Hannon TS, Saha CK, Carroll AE, et al. The ENCOURAGE healthy families study: A comparative effectiveness trial to reduce risk for type 2 diabetes in mothers and children. *Pediatr Diabetes.* 20 May 2018 [Epub ahead of print]
20. Foster GD, Linder B, Baranowski T, et al.; HEALTHY Study Group. A school-based intervention for diabetes risk reduction. *N Engl J Med* 2010;363:443–453
21. Bardenheier BH, Cogswell ME, Gregg EW, et al. Does knowing one's elevated glycemic status make a difference in macronutrient intake? *Diabetes Care* 2014;37:3143–3149
22. Hood MS, Little JP, Tarnopolsky MA, et al. Low-volume interval training improves muscle oxidative capacity in sedentary adults. *Med Sci Sports Exerc* 2011;43:1849–1856
23. Petrella AFM, Belfry G, Heath M. Older adults elicit a single-bout post-exercise executive benefit across a continuum of aerobically supported metabolic intensities. *Brain Res* 2019;1712:197–206
24. Tucker LA. Physical activity and telomere length in U.S. men and women: an NHANES investigation. *Prev Med* 2017;100:145–151
25. Pate RR, Pratt M, Blair SN, et al. Physical activity and public health: recommendation from the Centers for Disease Control and Prevention and the American College of Sports Medicine. *JAMA* 1995;273:402–407
26. Kimm SY, Glynn NW, Kriska AM, et al. Decline in physical activity in black and white girls during adolescence. *N Engl J Med* 2002;347: 709–715

27. Troiano RP, Berrigan D, Dodd KW, et al. Physical activity in the United States measured by accelerometer. *Med Sci Sports Exerc* 2008;40:181–188
28. Pettee Gabriel K, Sternfeld B, Colvin A, et al. Physical activity trajectories during midlife and subsequent risk of physical functioning decline in late mid-life: the Study of Women's Health Across the Nation (SWAN). *Prev Med* 2017;105:287–294
29. Vieira de Sousa M, Fukui R, Krustrup P, et al. Combination of recreational soccer and caloric restricted diet reduces markers of protein catabolism and cardiovascular risk in patients with type 2 diabetes. *J Nutr Health Aging* 2017;21:180–186
30. Eriksson KF, Lindgarde F. Prevention of type 2 (non-insulin-dependent) diabetes mellitus by diet and physical exercise: the 6-year Malmö feasibility study. *Diabetologia* 1991;34:891–898
31. Wadden TA, West DS, Neiberg RH, et al. One-year weight losses in the Look AHEAD study: factors associated with success. *Obesity (Silver Spring)* 2009;17:713–722
32. Wadden TA, Neiberg RH, Wing RR, et al. Four-year weight losses in the Look AHEAD study: factors associated with long-term success. *Obesity (Silver Spring)* 2011;19:1987–1998
33. Tate DF, Jackvony EH, Wing RR. Effects of Internet behavioral counseling on weight loss in adults at risk for type 2 diabetes: a randomized trial. *JAMA* 2003;289:1833–1836
34. Tate DF, Wing RR, Winett RA. Using Internet technology to deliver a behavioral weight loss program. *JAMA* 2001;285:1172–1177
35. Harvey-Berino J, Pintauro SJ, Buzzell P, et al. Does using the Internet facilitate the maintenance of weight loss? *Int J Obes* 2002;26:1254–1260
36. Wing RR, Tate DF, Gorin AA, et al. A self-regulation program for maintenance of weight loss. *N Engl J Med* 2006;355:1563–1571
37. Watson S, Woodside JV, Ware LJ, et al. Effect of a web-based behavior change program on weight loss and cardiovascular risk factors in overweight and obese adults at high risk of developing cardiovascular disease: randomized controlled trial. *J Med Internet Res* 2015;17:e177
38. Dening J, Islam SMS, George E, Maddison R. Web-based interventions for dietary behavior in adults with type 2 diabetes: systematic review of randomized controlled trials. *J Med Internet Res* 2020;22:e16437
39. Neve M, Morgan PJ, Jones PR, Collins CE. Effectiveness of web-based interventions in achieving weight loss and weight loss maintenance in overweight and obese adults: a systematic review with meta-analysis. *Obes Rev* 2010;11:306–321
40. Kodama S, Saito K, Tanaka S, et al. Effect of web-based lifestyle modification on weight control: a meta-analysis. *Int J Obes (Lond)* 2012;36:675–685

41. Baer HJ, Rozenblum R, De La Cruz BA, et al. Effect of an online weight management program integrated with population health management on weight change: a randomized clinical trial. *JAMA* 2020;324:1737–1746
42. Turk MW, Yang K, Hravnak M, et al. Randomized clinical trials of weight loss maintenance: a review. *J Cardiovasc Nurs* 2009;24:58–80
43. Camelon KM, Hådell K, Jämsén PT, et al. The Plate Model: a visual method of teaching meal planning. DAIS Project Group. Diabetes Atherosclerosis Intervention Study. *J Am Diet Assoc* 1998;98:1155–1158
44. Department of Agriculture Center for Nutrition Policy and Promotion. Dietary Guidelines for Americans. Available from https://www.myplate.gov/ Accessed 13 May 2021
45. Esposito K, Pontillo A, Di Palo C, et al. Effect of weight loss and lifestyle changes on vascular inflammatory markers in obese women: a randomized trial. *JAMA* 2003;289:1799–1804
46. Salas-Salvadó J, Guasch-Ferré M, Lee C-H, et al. Protective effects of the Mediterranean Diet on type 2 diabetes and metabolic syndrome. *J Nutr* 2015;146:920S–927S
47. Mozaffarian D, Marfisi R, Levantesi G, et al. Incidence of new-onset diabetes and impaired fasting glucose in patients with recent myocardial infarction and the effect of clinical and lifestyle risk factors. *Lancet* 2007;370:667–675
48. Esposito K, Maiorino MI, Bellastella G, et al. A journey into a Mediterranean diet and type 2 diabetes: a systematic review with meta-analyses. *BMJ Open* 2015;5:e008222
49. Gabel K, Hoddy KK, Haggerty N, et al. Effects of 8-hour time restricted feeding on body weight and metabolic disease risk factors in obese adults: a pilot study. *Nutr Healthy Aging* 2018;4:345–353
50. Ibrahim M, Al Magd MA, Annabi FA, et al. Recommendations for management of diabetes during Ramadan: update 2015. *BMJ Open Diabetes Res Care* 2015;3:e000108
51. Kalra S, Bajaj S, Gupta Y, et al. Fasts, feasts and festivals in diabetes-1: glycemic management during Hindu fasts. *Indian J Endocr Metab* 2015;19:198–203
52. Sarri KO, Tzanakis NE, Linardakis MK, et al. Effects of Greek Orthodox Christian Church fasting on serum lipids and obesity. *BMC Public Health* 2003;3:16
53. Mattson MP, Wan R. Beneficial effects of intermittent fasting and caloric restriction on the cardiovascular and cerebrovascular systems. *J Nutr Biochem* 2005;16:129–137
54. Anson RM, Guo Z, De Cabo R, et al. Intermittent fasting dissociates beneficial effects of dietary restriction on glucose metabolism and neuronal

resistance to injury from calorie intake. *Proc Natl Acad Sci U S A* 2003;100:6216–6220

55. Sundfør TM, Svendsen M, Tonstad S. Effect of intermittent versus continuous energy restriction on weight loss, maintenance and cardiometabolic risk: a randomized 1-year trial. *Nutr Metabo Cardiovasc Dis* 2018;28:698–706
56. Carter S, Clifton PM, Keogh JB. Effect of intermittent compared with continuous energy restricted diet on glycemic control in patients with type 2 diabetes: a randomized noninferiority trial. *JAMA Netw Open* 2018;1: e180756
57. Corley BT, Carroll RW, Hall RM, et al. Intermittent fasting in type 2 diabetes mellitus and the risk of hypoglycaemia: a randomized controlled trial. *Diabet Med* 2018;35:588–594
58. Li C, Sadraie B, Steckhan N, et al. Effects of a one-week fasting therapy in patients with type-2 diabetes mellitus and metabolic syndrome: a randomized controlled explorative study. *Exp Clin Endocrinol Diabetes* 2017;125:618–624
59. Ganesan K, Habboush Y, Dagogo-Jack S. Calorie restriction and intermittent fasting: impact on glycemic control in people with diabetes. *Diabetes Spectr* 2020;33:143–148
60. Lee CJ, Sears CL, Maruthur N. Gut microbiome and its role in obesity and insulin resistance. *Ann N Y Acad Sci* 2020;146:37–52
61. Crujeiras AB, Parra D, Goyenechea E, Martínez JA. Sirtuin gene expression in human mononuclear cells is modulated by caloric restriction. *Eur J Clin Invest* 2008;38:672–678
62. Wing RR, Phelan S. Long-term weight loss maintenance. *Am J Clin Nutr* 2005;82(Suppl.):222S–225S
63. Butryn ML, Phelan S, Hill JO, Wing RR. Consistent self-monitoring of weight: a key component of successful weight loss maintenance. *Obesity (Silver Spring)* 2007;15:3091–3096
64. Blonde L, Ginsberg BH, Horn S, et al. Frequency of blood glucose monitoring in relation to glycemic control in patients with type 2 diabetes. *Diabetes Care* 2002;25:245–246
65. Blonde L, Karter AJ. Current evidence regarding the value of self-monitored blood glucose testing. *Am J Med* 2005;118(Suppl. 9A): 20S–26S
66. Icek A. Perceived behavioral control, self-efficacy, locus of control, and the theory of planned behavior. *J Appl Soc Psychol* 2002;32:665–683
67. Hamilton K, White KM. Extending the theory of planned behavior: the role of self and social influences in predicting adolescent regular moderate-to-vigorous physical activity. *J Sport Exerc Psychol* 2008;30:56–74

68. Hamman RF, Wing RR, Edelstein SL, et al. Effect of weight loss with lifestyle intervention on risk of diabetes. *Diabetes Care* 2006;29:2102–2107
69. McAuley PA, Artero EG, Sui X, et al. Fitness, fatness, and survival in adults with prediabetes. *Diabetes Care* 2014;37:529–536
70. Johnson JL, Slentz CA, Ross LM, et al. Ten-year legacy effects of three eight-month exercise training programs on cardiometabolic health parameters. *Front Physiol* 2019;10:452
71. Miyatake N, Wada J, Kawasaki Y, et al. Relationship between metabolic syndrome and cigarette smoking in the Japanese population. *Intern Med* 2006;45:1039–1043
72. Facchini FS, Hollenbeck CB, Jeppesen J, et al. Insulin resistance and cigarette smoking. *Lancet* 1992;339:1128–1130
73. Heizer T, Yla-Herttuala S, Luoma J, et al. Cigarette smoking potentiates endothelial dysfunction of forearm resistance vessels in patients with hypercholesterolemia: role of oxidized LDL. *Circulation* 1996;9: 1346–1353
74. Kong C, Nimmo L, Elatrozy T, et al. Smoking is associated with increased hepatic lipase activity, insulin resistance, dyslipidaemia and early atherosclerosis in type 2 diabetes. *Atherosclerosis* 2001;156:373–378
75. Yeh H-C, Duncan BB, Schmidt MI, et al. Smoking, smoking cessation, and risk for type 2 diabetes mellitus: a cohort study. *Ann Intern Med* 2010;152:10–17
76. Oba S, Noda M, Waki K, et al.; Japan Public Health Center-Based Prospective Study Group. Smoking cessation increases short-term risk of type 2 diabetes irrespective of weight gain: the Japan Public Health Center-based Prospective Study. *PLoS One* 2012;7:e17061
77. Hu Y, Zong G, Liu G, et al. Smoking cessation, weight change, type 2 diabetes, and mortality. *N Engl J Med* 2018;379:623–632
78. Albright AL, Gregg EW. Preventing type 2 diabetes in communities across the U.S.: the National Diabetes Prevention Program. *Am J Prev Med* 2013;44(4 Suppl. 4):S346–S351
79. Echouffo-Tcheugui JB, Dagogo-Jack S. Preventing diabetes mellitus in developing countries. *Nat Rev Endocrinol* 2012;8:557–562
80. Herman WH, Hoerger TJ, Brandle M, et al.; Diabetes Prevention Program Research Group. The cost-effectiveness of lifestyle modification or metformin in preventing type 2 diabetes in adults with impaired glucose tolerance. *Ann Intern Med* 2005;142:323–332
81. Diabetes Prevention Program Research Group. The 10-year cost-effectiveness of lifestyle intervention or metformin for diabetes prevention: an intent-to-treat analysis of the DPP/DPPOS. *Diabetes Care* 2012; 35:723–730

82. Ramachandran A, Snehalatha C, Yamuna A, et al. Cost-effectiveness of the interventions in the primary prevention of diabetes among Asian Indians: within-trial results of the Indian Diabetes Prevention Programme (IDPP). *Diabetes Care* 2007;30:2548–2552
83. Ackermann RT, Marrero DG, Hicks KA, et al. An evaluation of cost sharing to finance a diet and physical activity intervention to prevent diabetes. *Diabetes Care* 2006;29:1237–1241

The Medicare Diabetes Prevention Program

In 2016, the Centers for Medicare and Medicaid Services made an important ruling that would make diabetes prevention services for Medicare patients reimbursable from 2018 onwards.[1,2] Besides the obvious personal health benefits, there is a strong economic rationale behind the decision to cover Medicare patients for diabetes prevention services. In reaching that decision, the Centers for Medicare and Medicaid Services noted that diabetes affects >25% of Americans aged 65 years or older (the Medicare-eligible population), and its prevalence is projected to increase approximately two-fold for all U.S. adults (ages 18–79 years) by 2050 if current trends continue. Medicare beneficiaries with diabetes consumed $42 billion more in health care costs in 2016 than beneficiaries who did not have diabetes.[1–4] The capitated costs per beneficiary showed that Medicare spent an estimated $1,500 more on Part D prescription drugs, $3,100 more for hospital and facility services, and $2,700 more in physician and other clinical services for people with diabetes than for people without diabetes.[1–4]

The Centers for Medicare and Medicaid Services' decision to cover diabetes prevention services, preferably delivered by trained layperson workers, creates a unique opportunity for the ~40% of the Medicare-eligible population who are at increased risk for diabetes/prediabetes. Because no drug has been approved by the U.S. Food and Drug Administration for prevention of diabetes, the only reimbursable approach is lifestyle counseling that results in weight loss of at least 5%, the threshold demonstrated to reduce diabetes risk in clinical trials.[1–5] The commercial health insurance industry tends to follow standards set by the Centers for Medicare and Medicaid Services, and it is anticipated that coverage for diabetes prevention services may soon be extended beyond Medicare patients. One concern is that the authority invoked by the Centers for Medicare and Medicaid Services in the 2016 decision to expand coverage for diabetes prevention was codified under Section 1115A(c) of the Affordable Care Act of 2010, a legislation that has repeatedly been under the threat of repeal by some politicians.

The Medicare Diabetes Prevention Program model is a structured intervention based on the Centers for Disease Control and Prevention (CDC)-approved curriculum.[3] The CDC curriculum is divided into a "core" phase and a "maintenance" phase. The core phase consists of 16 1-h intensive sessions over 6 months, delivered in a group-based format that provides practical training in long-term dietary change, increased physical activity, and behavior-change strategies for weight control. After the core sessions, less intensive follow-up meetings furnished monthly help ensure that the participants maintain healthy behaviors. The primary goal is at least 5% average weight loss by participants. Laypersons trained and certified in diabetes prevention counseling protocol by CDC-accredited entities are

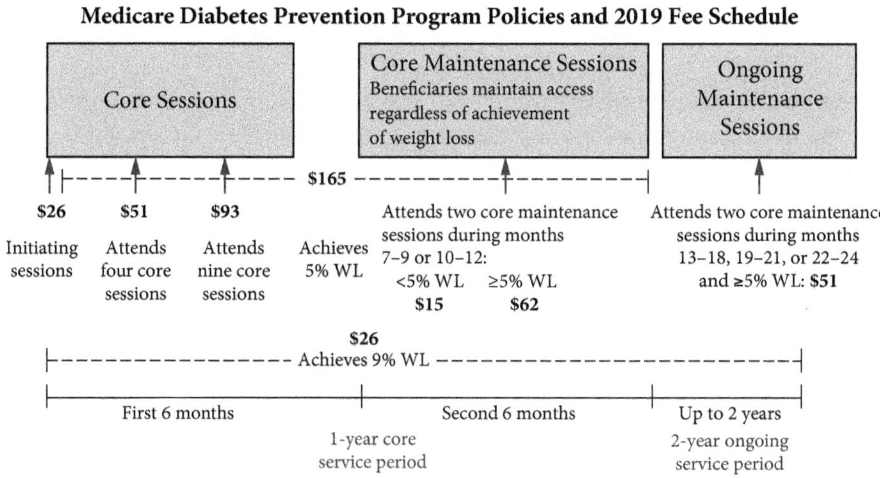

Figure 9.3—Summary of expectations and 2019 reimbursement schedule for the Medicare Diabetes Prevention Program. WL, weight loss.

specifically recommended to serve as lifestyle coaches. The approximate cost of such training and certification is $500.[3,4] The Centers for Medicare and Medicaid Services does not require the use of doctors, nurses, dietitians, or other trained professionals for delivery of lifestyle coaching.

The expectations and Medicare payment schedule are summarized in Fig. 9.3. The fees quoted are for 2019 and might be adjusted in future years.[5] The Centers for Medicare and Medicaid Services also offers a one-time "bridge payment" ($26 in 2019) to providers of diabetes prevention services when a beneficiary begins receiving services from them as a transfer from a different Medicare Diabetes Prevention Program provider.[5] The total payment can be up to ~$700 per prediabetic patient over 2 years, depending on completion of scheduled visits and achievement of target weight loss.[5] Although questions have been raised regarding the adequacy of the reimbursement for diabetes prevention services, the Medicare Diabetes Prevention Program is a significant step in the right direction, since it represents for the first time ever that diabetes prevention counseling has specifically attracted financial payment. The Medicare Diabetes Prevention Program also can serve as a catalyst for actualizing the idea of establishing freestanding Community Diabetes Prevention Centers. The economic viability of community diabetes prevention services depends to a large extent on the volume of individuals with prediabetes ("customers") that can be identified and referred to community programs.

Survey of Primary Care Physicians

Given the key role of primary care physicians as gatekeepers, a survey was conducted to gauge their interest in either setting up diabetes prevention services or referring eligible patients with prediabetes to obtain such services elsewhere. A one-page, five-item questionnaire was mailed to all 125 physician practices listed under Internal Medicine and Family Medicine sections of the membership roll of the Memphis Medical Society. The anonymous survey was mailed on 19 May 2017, and responses were received over a period of 7 days (earliest returns) to 66 days (last response received on 26 July 2017). A total of 38 primary care physicians responded to the survey, yielding a rate of 30.4%. The survey and results are presented in the sections that follow.

Survey Question 1: *"Approximately how many patients with diabetes do you see each month?"*

[ ] <10 [ ] 10–20 [ ] 20–40 [ ] >40

The purpose of this question was to gauge the exposure of primary care physicians to patients with diabetes. Because diabetes and prediabetes run in families, primary care physicians' diabetes volume likely would reflect access to a broader group of family members that potentially have prediabetes.

The pie chart and frequency distribution in Fig. 9.4 show that 50% of the responders indicated that they see >40 patients with diabetes each month. In addition to the 50% of responders who reported seeing >40 diabetes patients per month, 36.8% reported seeing 20–40 patients and 7.9% reported seeing 10–20 patients. Thus, ~95% of responders reported taking care of at least 10 diabetes patients per month.

Frequency distribution of diabetes patients/ year among primary care physicians

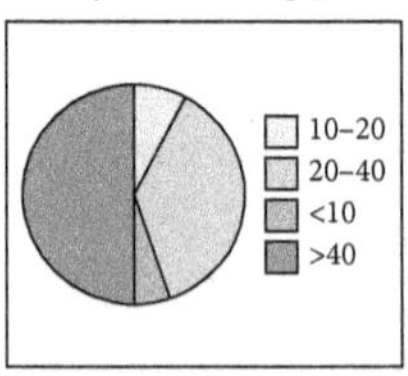

	Count	%
10–20	3	7.9
20–40	14	36.8
<10	2	5.3
>40	19	50.0
Total	38	100

Figure 9.4—Pie chart and frequency distribution data for survey question 1. The pie chart indicates how many diabetes patients responders see each month.

Distribution of prediabetes patients/ year among primary care physicians

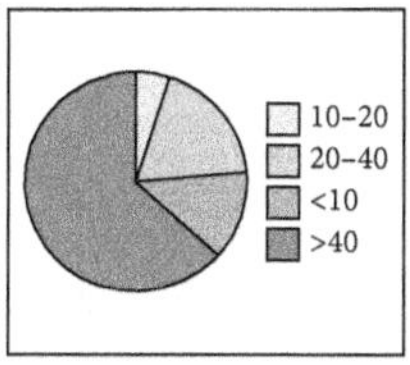

	Count	%
10–20	2	5.3
20–40	7	18.4
<10	5	13.2
>40	24	63.1
Total	38	100

Figure 9.5—Pie chart and frequency distribution data for survey question 2. The pie chart indicates how many diabetes patients responders see each month.

Survey Question 2: *"In the past year, approximately how many patients meeting criteria for prediabetes (i.e., fasting glucose 100–125 mg/dL, A1C 5.7–6.4%) have you seen in your practice?"*

[ ] <10 [ ] 10–20 [ ] 20–40 [ ] >40

As shown in the pie chart and frequency distribution in Fig. 9.5, 63.1% of the responders indicated that they see >40 patients with prediabetes each year.

In addition to the 63.1% of responders who reported seeing >40 prediabetes patients annually, 18.4% reported seeing 20–40 patients and 5.3% reported seeing 10–20 patients. Thus, ~87% of responders reported having access to at least 10 patients with prediabetes annually. A recent national survey of family physicians found that <1% of patients with laboratory tests consistent with prediabetes are diagnosed and treated for the condition; the overwhelming majority go undiagnosed.[6] Projecting from those national data, the actual numbers of individuals with prediabetes encountered by the responding Memphis physicians could be 100-fold higher than the numbers reported.

Survey Question 3: *"What is your usual approach when you find a patient meeting criteria for prediabetes?"*

[ ] Inform patient about result
[ ] Give general lifestyle advice
[ ] Refer to dietitian
[ ] Prescribe metformin
[ ] Other (Specify______________________________)

The purpose of this question is to assess the practice style of primary care physicians regarding management of patients with prediabetes. The responses are

Distribution of primary care physicians by number of prediabetes treatment modalities

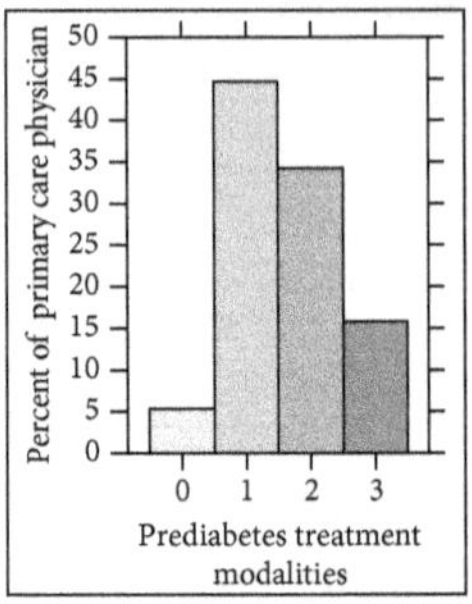

	Count	%
0	2	5.3
1	17	44.7
2	13	34.2
3	6	15.8
Total	38	100

Figure 9.6—Histogram and frequency distribution table in response to survey question 3.

converted to numerical scores, with 0 for no action besides informing the patient and 1 point for each of the treatment modalities (lifestyle advice, refer to dietitian, prescribe metformin).

As shown in the histogram and summarized in the frequency distribution table in Fig. 9.6, 44.7% of the responders indicated using one modality of treatment (usually lifestyle counseling), 34.2% reported using two modalities, and 15.8% used three treatment modalities (lifestyle advice, refer to dietitian, and prescribe metformin) for patients with prediabetes. Only 5.3% of primary care physicians indicated they do not offer any specific intervention for their patients with prediabetes. Twelve responders (31.6%) reported prescribing metformin along with lifestyle counseling, which is an off-label use of metformin. (Currently, the U.S. Food and Drug Administration [FDA] has not approved any medication for the treatment of prediabetes.) The percentage of primary care physicians who reported active intervention for prediabetes (nearly all responders) is considerably higher than data from a national survey of family physicians. In that survey, <1% of patients with lab tests showing prediabetes were diagnosed by primary care physicians and, among those who were diagnosed, only 35% had documentation of treatment targeted at prediabetes.[6] Although the possibility of social desirability bias[7,8] cannot be eliminated, the responses to survey question 4 do indicate a positive disposition of responders toward active intervention in patients with prediabetes.

Survey Question 4: *"Currently, no drug is FDA-approved for treating prediabetes, and diabetes prevention services are not readily reimbursed. Beginning in 2018, the Centers for Medicare and Medicaid Services may offer reimbursement for lifestyle intervention for diabetes prevention in Medicare patients delivered by trained personnel who*

have obtained certification by the CDC Diabetes Prevention Program. Reimbursement will be based on demonstrating at least 5% weight loss in patients enrolled in a clinic's Diabetes Prevention Program. Given this scenario, how likely are you to add trained personnel to your office to offer lifestyle diabetes prevention for Medicare patients?"

[ ] Very Likely   [ ] Likely   [ ] Neutral
[ ] Unlikely   [ ] Very Unlikely

The goal of this question is to get an estimate of the competition to be expected from primary care physicians in the future prediabetes market. As displayed in the frequency distribution table in Fig. 9.7, 34.2% of responders indicated they were very likely to add staff to enter the market, and 15.8% were likely to do so. Approximately 50% were undecided (neutral), unlikely, or very unlikely to enter the prediabetes market (see pie chart in Fig. 9.7).

Again, it is probable that the positive response rate was subject to social desirability bias, thereby overestimating the extent of potential competition.[8,9]

Likelihood of adding staff to enter the prediabetes market among primary care physicians

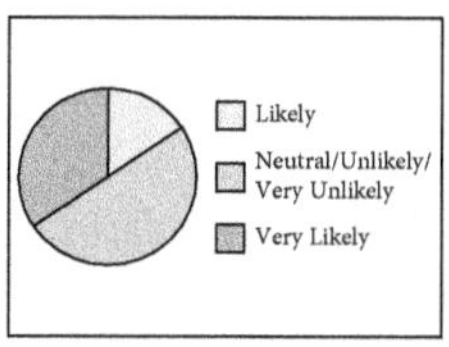

	Count	%
Likely	6	15.8
Neutral	9	23.7
Unlikely	6	15.8
Very Likely	13	34.2
Very Unlikely	4	10.5
Total	38	100

Figure 9.7—Pie chart and frequency distribution data for survey question 4.

Survey Question 5: *"If a center is established and staffed with CDC-certified personnel to offer a specialized lifestyle Diabetes Prevention Program for Medicare and other patients with prediabetes, how likely are you to refer patients found to have prediabetes to the center?"*

[ ] Very Likely   [ ] Likely   [ ] Neutral
[ ] Unlikely   [ ] Very Unlikely

This final and most important question is an estimate of the likelihood of referrals from primary care physicians to a dedicated prediabetes management center. In all, 76.3% of responders indicated that they were likely or very likely to refer their patients with prediabetes to the Prediabetes Management Center (PMC). There was little hesitation in the responses (only three responders were neutral); some 15.8% of responders indicated that they were unlikely or very unlikely to

Likelihood of referring prediabetes patients to a prediabetes management center among primary care physicians

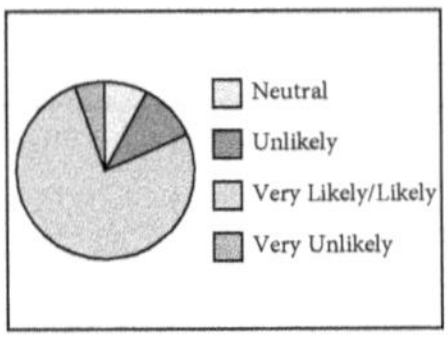

	Count	%
Likely	14	36.8
Neutral	3	7.9
Unlikely	4	10.5
Very Likely	15	39.5
Very Unlikely	2	5.3
Total	38	100

Figure 9.8—Pie chart and frequency distribution data for survey question 5.

refer patients to a dedicated prediabetes management center. These data are shown in the pie chart and frequency table in Fig. 9.8.

Comparing the responses to survey questions 4 and 5, it is interesting that whereas ~50% of primary care physicians indicated that they were likely or very likely to add staff to enter the prediabetes market (question 4), most of the primary care physicians (76.3%) also stated that they were likely or very likely to refer prediabetes patients to a local facility dedicated to diabetes prevention. This result suggests that at least half of the primary care physicians who were thinking of offering prediabetes management could decide to support a local diabetes prevention center instead of expanding their practice to cover that service.

Cautious generalizations from the survey

Because all members listed as practicing Internal Medicine or Family Medicine in the directory of membership of the Memphis Medical Society were mailed the survey, there was no element of selection bias. The ~30% response rate also is in the expected range for questionnaire surveys in social research. Table 9.4 summarizes

Table 9.4—Inferences from a Survey of Primary Care Physicians

- More than 50% of PCPs in Memphis have access to high volumes of patients with diabetes and prediabetes.
- 50% of PCPs in Memphis are unlikely to add prediabetes services, even with reimbursement for Medicare patients.
- 50% of PCPs in Memphis indicated that they are likely or very likely to enter a reimbursed prediabetes market.
- More than 75% of PCPs stated that they are likely or very likely to refer prediabetes patients to a dedicated diabetes prevention center for management.
- The prospect of multiple "Do-It-Yourself" diabetes prevention services being offered within PCP offices in Memphis seems unlikely.

PCP, primary care physician.

inferences from the primary care physicians' survey regarding prospects of offering or supporting diabetes prevention services directed at people with prediabetes.

Of course, Memphis is one city out of thousands in the world and the feedback from Memphis-based physicians cannot be generalized to other areas. Nonetheless, the survey data do provide some insight into likely physician behavior regarding support for a dedicated diabetes prevention center. As prediabetes is an asymptomatic condition, affected individuals usually feel relatively healthy and, given a choice, would likely prefer to receive preventive care at community-based centers instead of clinics and hospitals.

References

1. Centers for Medicare and Medicaid Services. Medicare Diabetes Prevention Program (MDPP) Expanded Model. Available from https://www.cms.gov/Newsroom/MediaReleaseDatabase/Fact-sheets/2016-Fact-sheets-items/2016-11-02-2.html Federal Register. Expansion of Medicare Diabetes Prevention Program Model. Available from https://www.federalregister.gov/documents/2016/11/15/ 2016-26668/med. Accessed 15 November 2020
2. Centers for Medicare and Medicaid Services. Medicare Diabetes Prevention Program (MDPP) Expanded Model. Available from https://innovation.cms.gov/innovation-models/medicare-diabetes-prevention-program. Accessed 15 November 2020
3. Centers for Disease Control and Prevention. National Diabetes Prevention Program. Available from www.cdc.gov/diabetes/prevention/recognition. Accessed 15 November 2020
4. Centers for Medicare and Medicaid Services. Medicare Diabetes Prevention Program (MDPP) Expanded Model. Available from https://go.cms.gov/mdpp. Accessed 15 November 2020
5. Centers for Medicare and Medicaid Services. Updating Calendar Year (CY) 2020 Medicare Diabetes Prevention Program (MDPP) Payment Rates. Available from https://www.cms.gov/Outreach-and-Education/Medicare-Learning-Network-MLN/MLNMattersArticles/Downloads/MM11455.pdf. Accessed 13 May 2021
6. Mainous AG, Tanner RJ, Baker R. Prediabetes diagnosis and treatment in primary care. *J Am Board Fam Med* 2016;29:283–285
7. Fisher RJ. Social desirability bias and the validity of indirect questioning. *Journal of Consumer Research* 1993;20:303–315
8. Fisher RJ, Katz JE. Social-desirability bias and the validity of self-reported values. Psychology & Marketing 2000;17(2):105–120. https://doi.org/10.1002/(SICI)1520-6793(200002)17:2<105::AID-MAR3>3.0.CO;2-9

Chapter 10

Exploratory Approaches to Prevent Type 2 Diabetes

Lifestyle Plus Cyclical Medication

The combination of lifestyle modification and medication has not been thoroughly examined. In the Indian Diabetes Prevention Program, neither low-dose metformin (Indian Diabetes Prevention Program-1) nor low-dose pioglitazone (Indian Diabetes Prevention Program-2) was additive to lifestyle modification for the outcome of diabetes prevention.[1,2] The reported relative diabetes risk reduction of ~28% with metformin in the Indian Diabetes Prevention Program-1 was comparable to the 31% reduction among metformin-treated subjects in the U.S.-based Diabetes Prevention Program, despite major differences in BMI and drug dosage (the Indian subjects were much leaner and received lower doses of metformin).[1,3] In the Indian Diabetes Prevention Program-2, the 3-year incidence of type 2 diabetes was comparable in the group treated with lifestyle modification alone and the group who received pioglitazone plus lifestyle modification. Trials of thiazolidinediones in other populations have shown effects on diabetes prevention that seemed more potent compared with the results observed in the Indian Diabetes Prevention Program-2.[4,5] Thus, the findings from the Indian Diabetes Prevention Program may be unique to the demographic group enrolled in those studies and do not eliminate the possibility of additive benefits from combined lifestyle plus medication intervention in other populations.

In the Actos Now for the Prevention of Diabetes (ACT NOW) trial that enrolled U.S. adults with prediabetes, treatment with pioglitazone resulted in a 72% diabetes risk reduction and a 48% conversion rate to normal glucose tolerance.[5] In the Canadian Normoglycemia Outcomes Evaluation (CANOE) trial, treatment with a combination of low doses of rosiglitazone and metformin showed a diabetes relative risk reduction of 66% and conversion to normal glucose regulation in 80% of participants.[6] Notably, the diabetes response rates to the thiazolidinedione drugs rosiglitazone and pioglitazone in terms of diabetes risk reduction in the U.S. and Canadian studies were numerically much higher than the ~30% rate reported in the Indian Diabetes Prevention Program.[3–6] Thus, there may be demographic differences in the response to some of the medications that have been tested for diabetes prevention. In a different study, the glucagon-like peptide 1 (GLP-1) receptor agonist liraglutide (3 mg daily) when added to lifestyle modification decreased the risk of incident type 2 diabetes by 79% compared with lifestyle modification alone in enrolled subjects with prediabetes.[7] Furthermore, 66% of participants assigned to liraglutide plus lifestyle modification reverted to normoglycemia compared with 36% of subjects in the group who received lifestyle modification alone.[7]

The medications tested for diabetes prevention so far have shown a loss of efficacy after being withdrawn. The newer sodium glucose–cotransporter-2 inhibitors induce weight loss and could potentially augment the effect of lifestyle intervention on diabetes prevention, but randomized controlled studies are lacking.

Although a purely drug-based approach to the prevention of type 2 diabetes is unattractive, for the reasons and limitations already discussed, a cyclical drug trial can be envisioned. Under this notion, combined lifestyle intervention and a selected medication is used to induce initial regression from prediabetes to normal glucose regulation, followed by withdrawal of drug and continuation of lifestyle intervention. Individuals are then followed for evidence of continued response or relapse from normal glucose regulation back to prediabetes during short- to mid-term (3- to 6-month) follow-up. Relapsers can be given a second cycle of medication superimposed on continued lifestyle intervention. Three or more such cycles could be tried before abandoning the regimen.

A study evaluating the merit of such a combined regimen comprising foundational lifestyle modification plus cyclical medication has not been reported. Based on the prediabetes regression data from the Diabetes Prevention Program, the initial restoration of normal glucose regulation under such a regimen could have a protective effect against long-term glycemic dysregulation. Because no drug is currently approved for treating people with prediabetes with the goal of preventing diabetes, any study along the proposed lines testing the off-label use of medications for diabetes prevention would require investigational new drug approval from the U.S. Food and Drug Association or an equivalent regulatory agency.

Designer Dietary and Nutraceutical Approaches

Unproven herbal and "natural" remedies are frequently touted for diabetes, and it is beyond the scope of this work to address those claims. Review of the emerging data on metabolomics suggests that elevations in circulating levels of certain amino acids are associated with increased risk of type 2 diabetes and prediabetes (discussed in Chapter 5). The list of such "diabetogenic" amino acids is lengthy, making their selective exclusion from a balanced diet nearly impossible as a strategy for diabetes prevention. Conversely, there have been several reports associating low levels of histidine and glycine with increased risks of type 2 diabetes and prediabetes.[8–10]

In a recent report from the Pathobiology of Prediabetes in a Biracial Cohort (POP-ABC) study, baseline plasma levels of aspartic acid plus asparagine and histidine were the only amino acids (out of 18 tested) that significantly predicted progression from normal glucose regulation to prediabetes. Each 1-SD increase in baseline aspartic acid and asparagine levels predicted a 2.72-fold higher risk of incident prediabetes, whereas a 1-SD increase in baseline histidine levels predicted a 10% lower risk of incident prediabetes.[10] Thus, it seems more feasible to design and test dietary or nutraceutical approaches that could prevent individuals with upper-normal glucose levels from breaking out into prediabetes. One example would be a preparation enriched with histidine and glycine and depleted of aspartic acid and asparagine.[11–13]

Preemptive Intervention in People at Risk of Drug-Induced Diabetes

Glucocorticoids and other medications can induce diabetes in some people receiving treatment for autoimmune or rheumatological disorders.[14] New-onset diabetes after transplantation is also a well-recognized entity.[15–18] The question often arises as to whether high-risk patients should receive prophylactic intervention to prevent diabetes before or concurrently with exposure to diabetogenic drugs (a form of "pharmacoprophylaxis"). Of course, referral for lifestyle modification should always be the initial strategy. However, many transplant patients may be too ill to practice effective lifestyle modification during the peri-transplant period. Patients in more stable clinical conditions receiving glucocorticoids or immunosuppressive agents for autoimmune or rheumatological disorders should be able to implement lifestyle modification to decrease their risk for drug-induced diabetes.

The 3-hydroxy-3-methylglutaryl–coenzyme A (HMG-CoA) reductase inhibitors (statins) are cholesterol-lowering drugs that are widely prescribed for primary and secondary prevention of atherosclerotic cardiovascular disease. Statin therapy was reported to increase the risk of treatment-emergent diabetes.[19–21] Although the association of statin therapy with increased diabetes risk is inconsistent,[22] some suggested mechanisms for the association include statin-induced weight gain, insulin resistance, and impaired insulin secretion.[23–25]

In 2012, the U.S. Food and Drug Administration added new safety label changes for the statin class of cholesterol-lowering drugs regarding the potential for increased A1C and fasting plasma glucose levels. Because statins are among the most widely consumed medications for cardioprotection, a balanced appraisal of the implications of their association with diabetes risk is warranted. Patients with established diabetes receiving statin medications may experience a modest to minimal increase in A1C levels (1.3 mmol/mol or 0.12%) compared with patients not treated with statins.[26]

The JUPITER study found an absolute difference of 0.6% in the risk of new cases of physician-diagnosed diabetes in patients assigned to rosuvastatin compared with placebo (3.0 vs. 2.4%). Ridker et al.[27] performed a risk/benefit analysis of the JUPITER study cohort, in which participants were stratified on the basis of having four major risk factors for developing diabetes: the metabolic syndrome, impaired fasting glucose, obesity (BMI >30 kg/m^2), or an A1C level of ≥6% at enrollment. The analysis showed that participants who harbored one or more of the four diabetes risk factors showed a 10.5-fold greater risk of developing diabetes during 5 years of follow-up compared with those who had none of the risk factors (incidence rate 1.88 vs. 0.18 per 100 person-years; hazard ratio 10.5 [95% CI 6.98–15.8]; $P = 0.001$).[27] The participants with one or more diabetes risk factors who had received rosuvastatin showed a 39% reduction in the primary end point (myocardial infarction, stroke, admission to hospital for unstable angina, arterial revascularization, or cardiovascular death), a 36% reduction in venous thromboembolism, a 17% reduction in total mortality, and a 28% increase in diabetes.[27] For participants with none of the major diabetes risk factors, statin treatment was associated with a 52% reduction in the primary end point, a 53% reduction in venous thromboembolism, a 22% reduction in total mortality, and no increase in diabetes.

Thus, despite their preexisting diabetes risk factors and the occurrence of treatment-emergent diabetes in the JUPITER trial, the participants who developed diabetes enjoyed cardiovascular risk reduction from statin therapy that was comparable to that seen in the entire study population.[19,27] Based on the available data, the benefits of statins clearly outweigh the risk of treatment-emergent diabetes. Furthermore, that risk can be predicted by assessing the presence of well-known diabetes risk factors (metabolic syndrome, impaired fasting glucose, obesity, and A1C ≥6%).[27] Thus, a careful documentation of diabetes and cardiometabolic risk factors along with blood glucose screening before initiation of statin therapy would seem reasonable as a risk mitigation strategy. Individuals harboring one or more of those risk factors, or people already known to have prediabetes, should be referred for lifestyle counseling for diabetes prevention as a general practice when considering statin therapy.

The concept of "pharmacoprophylaxis" is attractive and deserves to be formally tested in clinical trials. Should prophylactic treatment be initiated before, concurrently with, or after exposure to the known diabetogenic therapy? How long before, or how long after, exposure to a diabetogenic drug should the prophylactic intervention be started? Does the prophylactic treatment need to overlap completely with the duration of exposure to the diabetogenic therapy, or can evidence for more precise timing and duration be developed, based on pharmacokinetic and pharmacodynamics data? How often should blood glucose be monitored during pharmacoprophylaxis? And what else besides glucose should be monitored? Which medications would be most appropriate to consider for diabetes pharmacoprophylaxis? What criteria should be used for selecting patients for diabetes pharmacoprophylaxis? Should the selection criteria be based on the traditional risk factors of family history of diabetes, overweight/obesity, impaired fasting glucose, impaired glucose tolerance, hypertension, dyslipidemia, race/ethnicity, and history of gestational diabetes, or should specific factors related to transplantation (type and source of organ, immunosuppressive regimen, etc.) be considered?

Unfortunately, there is limited evidence-based information to answer these questions. Thus, randomized controlled studies are needed to demonstrate whether diabetes "pharmacoprophylaxis" is a rational strategy in high-risk individuals receiving treatment with potentially diabetogenic drugs. Obvious drug candidates for such randomized controlled trials would be metformin, thiazolidinediones, acarbose, and orlistat (all of which have been proven efficacious for diabetes prevention). Other agents, such as dipeptidyl peptidase-4 inhibitors, sodium glucose–cotransporter-2 inhibitors, and injectable and oral GLP-1 receptor agonists and the dopamine agonist bromocriptine-QR may be attractive trial candidates because of their low risk for iatrogenic hypoglycemia and interesting mechanisms of action.

Pragmatic patient selection for diabetes pharmacoprophylactic trials could include high-risk patients awaiting organ transplantation; patients about to receive prolonged high-dose steroid therapy for inflammatory, rheumatological, or other conditions; and patients receiving highly active antiretroviral therapy or antipsychotic agents who harbor diabetes risk factors (especially impaired fasting glucose or impaired glucose tolerance).[18,28–30] The benefits of prescribing any medications to prevent drug-induced diabetes must be balanced against adverse drug effects and costs. The reported adverse effects for the classes of potential agents include gastrointestinal disturbances (metformin, acarbose, orlistat, GLP-1 receptor agonists; lorcaserin phentermine/topiramate; naltrexone/bupropion); warning regarding pancreatitis (GLP-1 receptor agonist, dipeptidyl peptidase-4 inhibitors); special precautions in individuals with renal dysfunction (metformin, dipeptidyl peptidase-4 inhibitors, GLP-1 receptor agonist, sodium glucose–cotransporter-2 inhibitors); genital mycotic infections and ketoacidosis (sodium glucose–cotransporter-2 inhibitors); increased heart rate (GLP-1 receptor agonists); and multiple drug interactions, potential hypertensive crisis, and neuropsychiatric reactions (lorcaserin phentermine/topiramate, naltrexone/bupropion), among others.[18, 28-30]

In summary, the transplant recipients and patients receiving steroids and other agents face a significant risk of type 2 diabetes, and efforts to reduce that risk would be beneficial at the individual and societal levels. Whenever feasible, lifestyle intervention focusing on dietary and physical activity modifications should be initiated to prevent diabetes in high-risk individuals. Further studies are needed to develop specific lifestyle modification protocols tailored to the morbidity profiles of organ transplant recipients. Also, evidence-based data are needed to evaluate the concept of pharmacoprophylaxis for individuals about to receive exposure to potentially diabetogenic treatments.

Should Metabolic Surgery Be Used to Prevent Diabetes or Reverse Prediabetes?

Bariatric surgery induces massive weight loss (~25% to >95% depending on the study population, type of surgery, and length of follow-up).[31] Rapid resolution or marked attenuation of comorbid conditions, such as diabetes, hypertension, and dyslipidemia, has also been reported after bariatric surgery. Schauer et al.[32] randomized 150 patients with type 2 diabetes (age 49 ± 8 years, BMI ~37 kg/m^2, A1C 9.2%) to medical therapy, sleeve gastrectomy, or Roux-en-Y gastric bypass (RYGB) and assessed the effects on the primary outcome of attaining an A1C <6.0%.[32] After 1 year of follow-up, the mean weight loss was 5.4, 25.1, and 29.4 kg in patients assigned to medical therapy, sleeve gastrectomy, and RYGB, respectively. The proportion of patients attaining an A1C of <6.0% was 12, 42, and 37% in patients assigned to medical therapy, sleeve gastrectomy, and RYGB, respectively.[32] In another study of young to middle-aged patients (N = 60, BMI >35 kg/m^2, A1C 8.65%) randomized to medical therapy, gastric bypass, or biliopancreatic diversion, Mingrone et al.[33] reported that 95% of patients undergoing biliopancreatic diversion experienced remission of diabetes at 2 years. Diabetes remission was defined as a fasting plasma glucose level <100 mg/dL and an A1C level <6.5% for at least 1 year without drug therapy. The comparative diabetes remission rate was 75% for gastric bypass patients; no patient randomized to medical therapy experienced diabetes remission.[33]

In the Swedish Obese Subjects study, a nonrandomized, long-term follow-up study, bariatric surgery was associated with a 2-year diabetes remission rate of 72% (compared with 21% in a population control group of nonsurgically treated patients).[34] However, reassessment at 10 years showed a diabetes remission rate of 36% (versus 13% in control subjects).[34] A meta-analysis involving 621 studies, 888 treatment arms, and 135,246 patients concluded that bariatric procedures may be associated with complete clinical and biochemical resolution of diabetes in 78% of patients with type 2 diabetes.[35] Based on these and other supportive data, leading organizations have included metabolic surgery as a treatment option for adult patients with type 2 diabetes with BMI ≥40 kg/m^2 (≥37.5 kg/m^2 in Asian Americans) and patients with BMI of 35.0–39.9 kg/m^2 (32.5–37.4 kg/m^2 in Asian

Table 10.1—Comorbidities That May Lower the BMI Threshold for Recommending Metabolic Surgery in Obese Subjects[28]

• Type 2 diabetes
• Hypertension
• Obstructive sleep apnea
• Obesity-hypoventilation
• Pickwickian syndrome
• Nonalcoholic fatty liver disease
• Pseudotumor cerebri
• Gastroesophageal reflux disease
• Asthma
• Venous stasis disease
• Severe incontinence
• Debilitating arthritis
• Markedly impaired quality of life

Americans) who do not achieve durable weight loss and improvement in comorbidities with nonsurgical methods.[36,37] Metabolic surgery has also been suggested as an option for adolescents with type 2 diabetes with marked obesity (BMI >35 kg/m^2) refractory to lifestyle and pharmacological intervention, who have uncontrolled hyperglycemia and/or serious comorbidities.[38]

To date, there have been no recommendations for metabolic surgery to prevent diabetes. Neither prediabetes nor its component parts (impaired fasting glucose or impaired glucose tolerance) have been included in the long list of comorbidities that would make less than morbidly obese individuals without diabetes eligible for metabolic surgery[36–38] (Table 10.1). Data from the Swedish Obese Subjects study showed that among individuals who did not have diabetes at baseline, bariatric surgery was associated with a nearly 90% reduction (hazard ratio 0.22 [95% CI 0.18–0.27], $P < 0.001$) in the relative risk of incident type 2 diabetes during 15 years of postoperative follow-up.[39] The comparison group for that analysis was comprised of matched obese subjects in the community who were not necessarily following a Diabetes Prevention Program–type lifestyle intervention.[39]

Thus, the effect of surgery on incident diabetes among the Swedish cohort could have been overestimated. There is no doubt that metabolic surgery, through diverse mechanisms (including weight loss, improved insulin sensitivity, alterations in inflammatory cytokines, impact on metabolome and microbiome, etc.), would improve glucoregulation in obese people with prediabetes. However, the threshold weight loss required for diabetes prevention and possible regression to normal glucose regulation (~5–7%) in people with prediabetes is achievable by nonsurgical means. Despite advances in surgical techniques and postoperative care, bariatric surgery still carries finite risks, including peri-operative mortality.[40] Moreover, depending on the specific procedures, the cumulative burden of lifelong medical follow-up and management of macronutrient and micronutrient derangements could be significant, if metabolic surgery were undertaken strictly for diabetes prevention.[41] Of course, the counterargument is the promise of avoidance of premature mortality from morbid obesity that may be delivered by timely metabolic surgery.[42]

References

1. Ramachandran A, Snehalatha C, Mary S, et al. The Indian Diabetes Prevention Programme shows that lifestyle modification and metformin prevent type 2 diabetes in Asian Indian subjects with impaired glucose tolerance (IDPP-1). *Diabetologia* 2006;49:289–297
2. Ramachandran A, Snehalatha C, Mary S, et al. Pioglitazone does not enhance the effectiveness of lifestyle modification in preventing conversion of impaired glucose tolerance to diabetes in Asian Indians: results of the Indian Diabetes Prevention Programme-2 (IDPP-2). *Diabetologia* 2009;52:1019–1026
3. Knowler WC, Barret-Connor E, Fowler SE, et al.; Diabetes Prevention Program Research Group. Reduction in the incidence of type 2 diabetes with lifestyle intervention or metformin. *N Engl J Med* 2002;346:393–403
4. DREAM (Diabetes Reduction Assessment with Ramipril and Rosiglitazone Medication) Trial Investigators. Effect of rosiglitazone on the frequency of diabetes in patients with impaired glucose tolerance or impaired fasting glucose: a randomized controlled trial. *Lancet* 2006;368:1096–1105
5. DeFronzo RA, Tripathy D, Schwenke DC, et al.; ACT NOW Study. Pioglitazone for diabetes prevention in impaired glucose tolerance. *N Engl J Med* 2011;364:1104–1115
6. Zinman B, Stewart BH, Neuman J, et al. Low-dose combination therapy with rosiglitazone and metformin to prevent type 2 diabetes mellitus (CANOE trial): a double-blind randomized controlled study. *Lancet* 2010;376:103–111
7. Pi-Sunyer X, Astrup A, Fujioka K, et al.; SCALE Obesity and Prediabetes NN8022-1839 Study Group. A randomized, controlled trial of 3.0 mg of liraglutide in weight management. *N Engl J Med* 2015;373:11–22

8. Razak MA, Begum PS, Viswanath B, Rajagopal S. Multifarious beneficial effect of nonessential amino acid, glycine: a review. *Oxid Med Cell Longev* 2017;2017:1716701
9. Li X, Sun L, Zhang W, et al. Association of serum glycine levels with metabolic syndrome in an elderly Chinese population. *Nutr Metab (Lond)* 2018;15:89
10. Owei I, Umekwe U, Stentz F, et al. Amino acid signature predictive of incident prediabetes: a case-control study nested within the longitudinal pathobiology of prediabetes in a biracial cohort. *Metabolism* 2019;98: 76–83
11. Houjeghani S, Kheirouri S, Faraji E. L-carnosine supplementation attenuated fasting glucose, triglycerides, advanced glycation end products, and tumor necrosis factor–α levels in patients with type 2 diabetes: a double-blind placebo-controlled randomized clinical trial. *Nutr Res* 2018;49: 96–106
12. Lee YT, Hsu CC, Lin MH, et al. Histidine and carnosine delay diabetic deterioration in mice and protect human low density lipoprotein against oxidation and glycation. *Eur J Pharmacol* 2005;513:145–150
13. Liu Y, Cotillard A, Vatier C, et al. A dietary supplement containing cinnamon, chromium and carnosine decreases fasting plasma glucose and increases lean mass in overweight or obese pre-diabetic subjects: a randomized, placebo-controlled trial. *PLoS One* 2015;10:e0138646
14. Liu MZ, He HY, Luo JQ, et al. Drug-induced hyperglycaemia and diabetes: pharmacogenomics perspectives. *Arch Pharm Res* 2018;41: 725–736
15. Hjelmesaeth J, Hartmann A, Leivestad T, et al. The impact of early diagnosed new-onset post-transplantation diabetes mellitus on survival and major cardiac events. *Kidney Int* 2006;69:588–595
16. Lane JT, Dagogo-Jack S. Approach to the patient with new-onset diabetes after transplant (NODAT). *J Clin Endocrinol Metab* 2011;96:3289–3297
17. Gosmanov AR, Dagogo-Jack S. Predicting, managing and preventing new-onset diabetes after transplantation. *Minerva Endocrinol* 2012;37: 233–246
18. Dagogo-Jack S. *Diabetes Risks from Prescription and Nonprescription Drugs: Mechanisms and Approaches to Risk Reduction.* Alexandria, VA, American Diabetes Association, 2016

19. Ridker PM, Danielson E, Fonseca FAH, et al.; JUPITER Study Group. Rosuvastatin to prevent vascular events in men and women with elevated C-reactive protein. *N Eng J Med* 2008;359:2195–2207
20. Culver AL, Ockene IS, Balasubramanian R, et al. Statin use and risk of diabetes mellitus in postmenopausal women in the Women's Health Initiative. *Arch Intern Med* 2012;172:144–152
21. Sattar N, Preiss D, Murray HM, et al. Statins and risk of incident diabetes: a collaborative meta-analysis of randomised statin trials. *Lancet* 2010; 375:735–742
22. Rajpathak SW, Kumbhani DJ, Crandall J, et al. Statin therapy and risk of developing type 2 diabetes: a meta-analyses. *Diabetes Care* 2009;32: 1924–1929
23. Swerdlow DI, Preiss D, Kuchenbaecker KB, et al. HMG-coenzyme A reductase inhibition, type 2 diabetes, and bodyweight: evidence from genetic analysis and randomised trials. *Lancet* 2015;385: 351–361
24. Cederberg H, Stančáková A, Yaluri N, et al. Increased risk of diabetes with statin treatment is associated with impaired insulin sensitivity and insulin secretion: a 6 year follow-up study of the METSIM cohort. *Diabetologia* 2015;58:1109–1117
25. Sposito AC, Carvalho LSF, Moura FA, et al. Statin short-term inhibition of insulin sensitivity and secretion during acute phase of ST-elevation myocardial infarction. *Sci Rep* 2019;9:16401
26. Erqou S, Lee CC, Adler AI. Statins and glycaemic control in individuals with diabetes: a systematic review and meta-analysis. *Diabetologia* 2014;57:2444–2452
27. Ridker PM, Pradhan A, MacFadyen JG, et al. Cardiovascular benefits and diabetes risks of statin therapy in primary prevention: an analysis from the JUPITER trial. *Lancet* 2012;380:565–571
28. Dagogo-Jack S. New drugs and diabetes risk: antipsychotic and antiretroviral agents. In *Clinical Diabetes*. Fonseca VA, Ed. Philadelphia, Saunders, 2006, pp. 569–581
29. Dagogo-Jack S. HIV therapy and diabetes risk (Editorial). *Diabetes Care* 2008;31:1267–1268
30. Dagogo-Jack S. The role of antipsychotic agents in the development of diabetes. *Nat Clin Pract Endocrinol Metab* 2009;5:22–23

31. Bolen SD, Chang HY, Weiner JP, et al. Clinical outcomes after bariatric surgery: a 5-year matched cohort analysis in 7 US states. *Obes Surg* 2012;22:749–763
32. Schauer PR, Kashyap SR, Wolski K, et al. Bariatric surgery versus intensive medical therapy in obese patients with diabetes. *N Engl J Med* 2012;366:1567–1576
33. Mingrone G, Panunzi S, De Gaetano A, et al. Bariatric surgery versus conventional medical therapy for type 2 diabetes. *N Engl J Med* 2012;366: 1577–1585
34. Sjöström L, Lindroos A-K, Peltonen M, et al. Lifestyle, diabetes, and cardiovascular risk factors 10 years after bariatric surgery. *N Engl J Med* 2004;351:2683–2693
35. Buchwald H, Estok R, Fahrbach K, et al. Weight and type 2 diabetes after bariatric surgery: systematic review and meta-analysis. *Am J Med* 2009; 122:248–256.e5
36. American Diabetes Association. 8. Obesity management for the treatment of type 2 diabetes: *Standards of Medical Care in Diabetes—2020. Diabetes Care* 2020;43:S89–S97
37. Garvey WT, Mechanick JI, Brett EM, et al.; Reviewers of the AACE/ACE Obesity Clinical Practice Guidelines. American Association of Clinical Endocrinologists and American College of Endocrinology Comprehensive Clinical Practice Guidelines for Medical Care of Patients with Obesity. *Endocr Pract* 2016;22(Suppl. 3):1–203
38. American Diabetes Association. 13. Children and adolescents: *Standards of Medical Care in Diabetes—2020. Diabetes Care* 2020;43(Suppl. 1): S163–S182
39. Carlsson LMS, Peltonen M, Ahlin S, et al. Bariatric surgery and prevention of type 2 diabetes in Swedish obese subjects. *N Engl J Med* 2012;367:695–704
40. Cardoso L, Rodrigues D, Gomes L, Carrilho F. Short- and long-term mortality after bariatric surgery: a systematic review and meta-analysis. *Diabetes Obes Metab* 2017;19:1223–1232
41. Mesureur L, Arvanitakis M. Metabolic and nutritional complications of bariatric surgery: a review. *Acta Gastroenterol Belg* 2017;80:515–525
42. Arterburn DE, Olsen MK, Smith VA, et al. Association between bariatric surgery and long-term survival. *JAMA* 2015;313:62–70

Index

Note: Page numbers followed by an *f* refer to figures. Page numbers followed by a *t* refer to tables. Page numbers in **bold** indicate an in-depth discussion.

B

C

D

E

F

G

H

P

Q

R

S

T

About the Author

Sam Dagogo-Jack, MD, DSc, is Professor of Medicine and Chief of the Division of Endocrinology, Diabetes, and Metabolism at the University of Tennessee Health Science Center (UTHSC) in Memphis, where he holds the A.C. Mullins Endowed Professorial Chair in Translational Research. He is also Director of the General Clinical Research Center at UTHSC. Dr. Dagogo-Jack's current research focuses on the interaction of genetic and environmental factors in the pathobiology of prediabetes and prevention of diabetes. He is a past president, Medicine and Science, of the American Diabetes Association and a recipient of the Banting Medal for Leadership from the American Diabetes Association and the Distinction in Endocrinology Award from the American College of Endocrinology.

www.ingramcontent.com/pod-product-compliance
Lightning Source LLC
Jackson TN
JSHW070940111125
93945JS00003B/10